10 COMMANDMENTS OF HEART HEALTH
explained

Dr Warrick Bishop

and

Dr Karam Kostner

with

Penelope Edman

https://drwarrickbishop.com/s/pmi7d

10 COMMANDMENTS OF HEART HEALTH
explained

understanding the cause and prevention strategies to reduce your risk of one of the world's most prevalent killers

This book is for you, if you

- want to reduce your risk of a heart attack;
- believe that prevention is better than cure;
- come from a family with a history of 'bad' hearts;
- would enjoy an informative read about the main killer of our generation;
- are a medical, nursing or other health professional student looking for a 'taster' that puts you 'ahead of the game' in your learning;
- are a pro-active doctor seeking current information about risk and prevention;
- are a collaborative medico who recommends good, informative books to your patients.

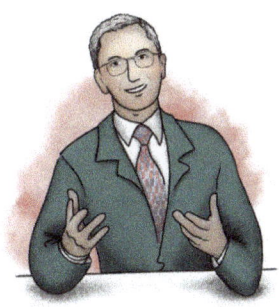

This book is for you if you have a heart.

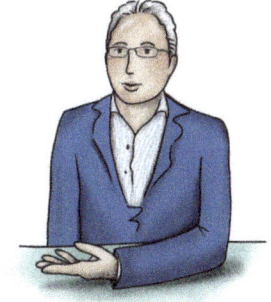

PUBLISHER'S NOTE

The authors and editors of this publication have made every effort to provide information that is accurate and complete as of the date of publication. Readers are advised not to rely on the information provided without consulting their own medical advisers. It is the responsibility of the reader's treating physician or specialist, who relies on experience and knowledge about the patient, to determine the condition of, and the best treatment for, the reader. The information contained in this publication is provided without warranty of any kind. The authors and editors disclaim responsibility for any errors, mis-statements, typographical errors or omissions in this publication.

© 2024 Warrick Bishop MBBS FRACP

This publication is copyright. Other than for the purposes of and subject to the conditions prescribed under the Copyright Act, no part of it may in any form or by any means (electronic, mechanical, micro-copying, photocopying, recording or otherwise) be reproduced, stored in a retrieval system or transmitted without prior written permission.

Any information reproduced herein which has been obtained from any other copyright owner has been reproduced with that copyright owner's permission but does not purport to be an accurate reproduction. Inquiries should be addressed to the publisher.

National Library of Australia Cataloguing-in-Publication entry

Authors:	Dr Warrick Bishop MBBS FRACP
	Dr Karam Kostner MD PhD FRACP FCSANZ
Writer:	Penelope Edman, PACE 56
Title:	10 Commandments of Heart Health Explained
	First Edition - 2024 - V5 - 250524
ASIN:	(Amazon Kindle)
ISBN:	978-0-9756310-3-4 (eBook)
ISBN:	978-0-9756310-4-1 (Amazon Paperback)
ISBN:	978-0-9756310-5-8 (Amazon Hardcover)
ISBN:	978-0-9756310-6-5 (Ingram Spark PAPERBACK)
ISBN:	978-0-9756310-7-2 (Ingram Spark HARDCOVER)
Subject:	Cardiac health care
Publisher:	Dr Warrick Bishop MBBS FRACP
Designer:	Cathy McAuliffe, *Cathy McAuliffe Design*
Illustrator:	Cathy McAuliffe, *Cathy McAuliffe Design*

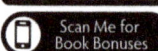

https://drwarrickbishop.com/s/pmi7d

*dedicated to
our Michelles,
for their ongoing love,
encouragement, and inspiration
as we promote heart health*

CONTENTS

about the authors 8
foreword 12
preface 15
introduction   good health and fitness are not guarantees for a healthy heart 17
                 patient's perspective – Dan 18
                 patient's perspective – Ron 22
                 patient's perspective – Darren 24

a healthy heart

chapter 1   the healthy heart 31
chapter 2   how does a heart attack happen? 41
                 answering your questions – what does a healthy artery look like? 42
                 answering your questions – what is cholesterol? 44
                 a closer look – formation of a clot 48
                 a closer look – heart attack and sudden cardiac arrest ... 51
chapter 3   being ahead of the game 55

10 commandments of heart health

chapter 4   the 10 commandments 67
chapter 5   quit! quit! quit! 77
chapter 6   body and mind 83
                 physical vitality 83
                 personal comment – heat shock proteins 86
                 mental well-being 87
chapter 7   obesity 95
                 a closer look – bariatric surgery 101
chapter 8   'what should I eat, doc?' 103
                 a closer look – please eat more veggies! 110
                 a closer look – not so simple carbohydrates 110
                 personal comment – the pleasure of wine 114
chapter 9   blood pressure – why the fuss? 117
                 answering your questions – is there a perfect BP? 122

chapter 10	blood sugar overload	127
	a closer look – new drugs	132
chapter 11	should we guess or take a look?	135
	patient's perspective – Conrad	138
	case study – Tracey and Beck	139
	case study – Tony	141
	case study – Penny (and her husband)	143
	a closer look – stress testing	150
	case study – Bill	152
chapter 12	dealing with cholesterol	155
	case study – John	157
	case study – Karen	158
chapter 13	aspirin – friend or foe?	163
chapter 14	teamwork	171
chapter 15	Dan *didn't* have a heart attack	175
	patient's perspective – Dan	176
	answering your questions – what is coronary artery bypass grafting?	178
	a closer look – ECMO	182
	patient's perspective – Ron	187
epilogue	life after death	193
appendices		
appendix 1	will you recognise your heart attack?	199
appendix 2	sobering statistics	200
appendix 3	swap this for that	202
appendix 4	surviving the odds: defibrillators save lives	203
	'what if?' leads to Heart 180	203
	second chance brings new passion	205
access to interviews and further information		210
references		212
glossary		213
index		227
acknowledgements and thanks		231

ABOUT THE AUTHORS

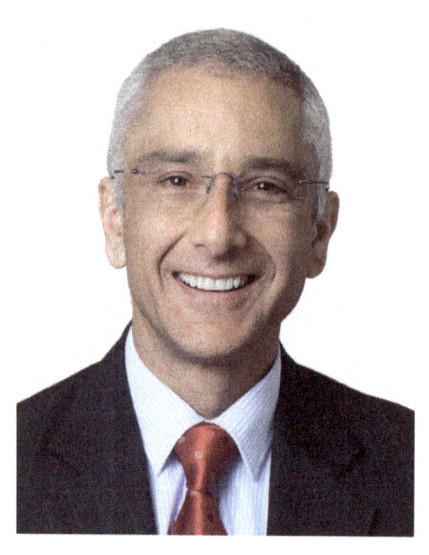

WARRICK BISHOP is a practicing cardiologist passionate about helping people live as well as possible for as long as possible. He is particularly interested in preventing heart attacks by using cardiac CT imaging, managing cholesterol, and giving attention to diet. He also supports patients through education, believing that the best-educated patients receive the best health care.

Warrick graduated from the University of Tasmania School of Medicine in 1988. He worked in the Northern Territory before undertaking specialist training in Adelaide, South Australia. He completed his advanced training in cardiology in Hobart, Tasmania, becoming a fellow of the Royal Australian College of Physicians in 1997. He has worked predominantly in private practice.

In 2009, Warrick undertook training in CT cardiac coronary angiography, becoming the first cardiologist in Tasmania with this specialist recognition. This area of imaging fits well with his interest in preventative cardiology and was the focus of his first book, *Have You Planned Your Heart Attack?* (2016). He is a member of the Society of Cardiovascular Computed Tomography, Australian and New Zealand International Regional Committee (SCCT ANZ IRC).

Warrick is also a member of the Australian Atherosclerosis Society and a participant on the panel of 'interested parties' developing a model of care and a national registry for familial hypercholesterolemia. He has also developed a particular interest in diabetic-related risk of coronary artery disease, allied explicitly to eating guidelines and lipid profiles.

Warrick is an accredited examiner for the Royal Australian College of Physicians and is regularly involved with teaching medical students and junior doctors. He has worked on projects, in an affiliate capacity, with Hobart's globally recognised Menzies Institute for Medical Research. He has academic status at the Medical School of the University of Tasmania.

As a member of the Clinical Issues Committee of the Australian Heart Foundation, which provides input into issues of significance for managing heart patients, Warrick contributed to the Australian Heart Foundation's 2021 position paper on Coronary Artery Calcium.

Warrick enjoys a strong social media profile. In February 2020, he presented a TEDx talk, *Lessons from a Heart Attack*, at Docklands, Victoria, Australia, and then another soon after, *How Medicine, Money and Mindset are Costing Lives*, before a live audience at the University of Mississippi, Jackson, Mississippi, USA.

In addition to authoring numerous articles and books, *Have You Planned Your Heart Attack?* (published in the USA as *Know Your Real Risk of Heart Attack*), *Atrial Fibrillation Explained, Cardiac Failure Explained, Cardiac Rehabilitation Explained,* and now *10 Commandments of Heart Health Explained*, he founded the Healthy Heart Network in 2018.

This book, with Dr Karam Kostner of Brisbane, Queensland, is his second collaborative venture. The first, *Cardiac Rehabilitation Explained*, was with fellow cardiologist Dr Alistair Begg of Adelaide, South Australia.

Warrick focuses all his public endeavours on helping people live as well as possible for as long as possible through education and support.

He is a keen intermittent faster who values family and friends, music, travel and keeping himself as well as possible for as long as possible.

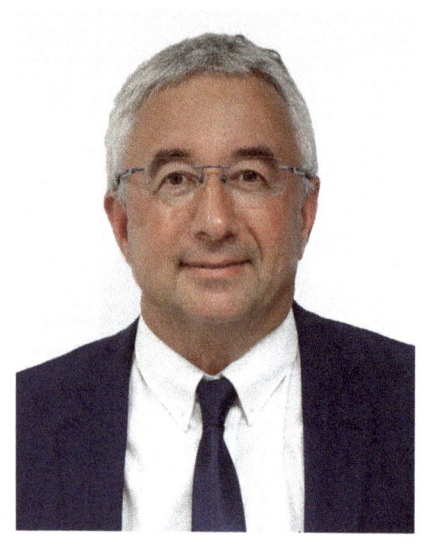

KARAM KOSTNER is an Associate Professor of Medicine at the University of Queensland and Director of Cardiology at Mater Public and Private Hospitals in Brisbane. As a cardiologist and one of the most experienced lipidologists in Australia, he oversees a large public and private lipid clinic. He is also a director of Cholesterol Care Australia, a specialist cholesterol clinic and research facility in Brisbane and a senior cardiologist with Heart of Australia, which delivers specialist healthcare services and testing to rural, remote, and indigenous communities across Queensland.

Karam's clinical interests are preventative cardiology and lipid disorders. His passion combines helping people with high cholesterol and investigating new therapies for patients with elevated cholesterol. Cardiovascular research has involved him for 20 years, and, as principal investigator, he has conducted more than 65 clinical trials including many trials on lipid lowering therapies. His team developed an extracorporeal lipid removal technique called lipid apheresis and the first patients worldwide were trialled by his team in Brisbane. The team also developed a medication to decrease lipoprotein (a) which is currently in clinical trials.

Karam completed his schooling and most of his medical studies in Austria. He undertook post-doctoral work at the Royal Brisbane Hospital, University of Queensland, Brisbane (1991-93) before returning to Austria where he undertook specialty training in internal medicine (1994-98), graduating as a specialist in Internal Medicine in December 1998, before undertaking speciality training in cardiology (1998-2000), becoming a specialist cardiologist in March 2001. He became a professor of medicine in Austria at the age of 33 and is currently an Associate Professor of Medicine at the University of Queensland. He returned to Australia in 2001 settling in Brisbane and continuing his career at the Mater Hospital and UQ.

Government and medical bodies regularly consult Karam about approval of and funding for new and established lipid-lowering therapies.

Having published more than 100 peer-reviewed papers, four book chapters and several review articles and editorials, Karam has also delivered numerous invited lectures at cardiovascular meetings and is past president of the Cardiac Society of Australia and NZ, Queensland branch. Currently, he is an associate editor of *Atherosclerosis* and *The Journal of Preventive Cardiology* and an associate editor and cardiovascular section editor of the *European Journal Clinical Investigation* (a peer-reviewed medical journal that covers a wide range of clinical research and investigations in various fields of medicine) and a regular reviewer for many journals, as well as being a National Health and Medical Research grant reviewer. (The NHMR is the leading body for health and medical research in Australia, responsible for providing funding, setting guidelines, and promoting research excellence in health and medicine.)

Karam has also organised, or been on the committee of, several national and international conferences and has been the chair and organiser of the World Congress of Clinical Lipidology on three occasions.

Outside of work Karam loves outdoor activities such as skiing and hiking with his family and friends and is a very keen fisherman.

FOREWORD

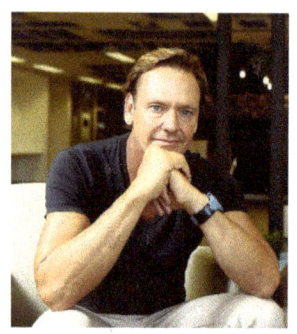

In a world where we often push ourselves to the limit, chasing our dreams and ambitions, we can easily forget to prioritise one thing that truly matters – our heart health.

It was a wake-up call for me when I lost one of my closest mates, Chucky, to a heart incident on the beach after we had finished a paddle fitness class together. That tragedy was a stark reminder that none of us is invincible, no matter how fit or strong we may feel. It led me on a journey to understand and promote heart health, especially the need for more automated external defibrillators (AEDs) in the community.

I'm thrilled to introduce you to *10 Commandments of Heart Health Explained*, a book that encapsulates the essence of this journey. Authored by renowned cardiologist Dr Warrick Bishop and esteemed lipidologist Dr Karam Kostner, this book is a beacon of hope and a roadmap to a healthier heart.

Throughout these pages, you'll find a wealth of knowledge distilled from the combined expertise and dedication of these two committed and caring medical professionals. They've made it their life's work to demystify the complexities of heart health, breaking it down into 10 crucial 'commandments' that form the foundation of a heart-healthy lifestyle.

Not long after Chucky's death, I insisted that about 100 of my mates undergo heart screening. The results were astonishing. Each was a 'fit and healthy' individual, aged between 39 and 72. As a result of these check-ups, five people needed stents, while another 15 needed to start taking medication. Discovering potential issues early allowed them to take proactive steps towards better heart health. It was a real eye-opener!

The wisdom contained within these pages will help you understand the complexities of the heart. From the importance of cholesterol to embracing exercise, from nourishing your body to managing stress, this book covers it all! Dr Bishop and Dr Kostner have a gift for sharing complex medical concepts in a practical and actionable way that anyone can follow.

Each 'commandment' is not a suggestion but a call to action.

By incorporating these principles into your life as early as possible, you're not only prolonging your years but also enhancing the quality of life of those years. You're giving yourself the gift of vitality and resilience – and the ability to chase your dreams with a heart that beats strong and true.

So, I encourage you to dive into the wisdom within these pages. Embrace the 'commandments'. Make them a part of your daily routine. Watch as they transform not just your heart but your life.

Together, let's champion heart health – for ourselves and those we hold dear.

Here's to a healthier, happier heart!

GUY LEECH

Founder/CEO of Heart180

world and Australian Ironman champion

world and Australian Paddleboard champion

dubbed the 'fittest man in Australia' by the Australian Institute of Sport (1993)

winner of the television reality show
I'm a Celebrity. Get Me Out of Here: Vanuatu *(2006)*

UNLOCK THE FULL POTENTIAL OF YOUR READING EXPERIENCE WITH EXCLUSIVE ACCESS TO OUR SPECIAL BOOK BONUSES!

Dive deeper into the vital topic of heart health with our carefully curated selection of bonus materials, designed to complement your journey through the pages.

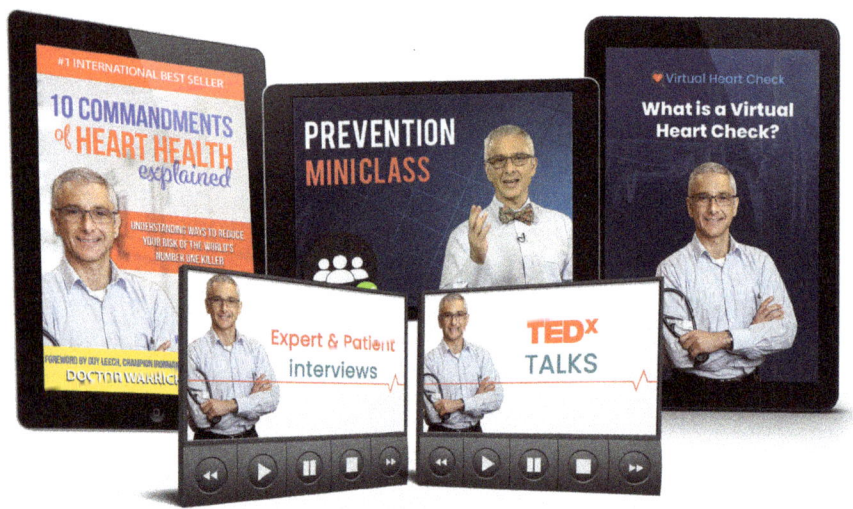

10 Commandments of Heart Health Explained
book bonuses
https://drwarrickbishop.com/s/pmi7d

PREFACE

As cardiologists, we have met very few patients who expected to have a heart problem. Patients do not put in their diaries "possible problem with my heart next week".

Yet, what if we could be forewarned about, or prepared for, a potential problem with our coronary arteries? What if we could take away the surprise – the emergency – of a heart attack occurring 'out of the blue' and replace possible fear with prepared understanding and a preventative lifestyle? What if we could live proactively to minimise the risk of having a heart attack?

Current thinking about a heart attack focuses on the **emergency**. The **response** to that emergency is the *chain of survival*. However, that can be too late.

We want to reframe community thinking, broadening the conversation to *a loop of life*. This means that our focus extends beyond the victim of a heart attack to enquire if there are other family members who could be at risk ... friends who could be at risk ... responders who could be at risk ... and so the loop expands to *all who could be at risk*.

We might have the services of top-notch tow truck operators available to us, but surely the most prudent option is to avoid the breakdown ... the accident ... the emergency ... in the first place!

All heart attacks are emergencies, traumatic, and incur huge costs (well beyond money). **Most** heart attacks are preventable.

What if we could **plan** NOT to have a heart attack?

This book details how you, the reader, can have a starring role in making that happen. Be aware. Know and understand your risks. Take preventative action. Follow our *10 Commandments*.

Dr Warrick Bishop (Hobart), *Dr Karam Kostner* (Brisbane)

上医医未病之病
中医医将病之病
下医医已病之病
～黄帝内经～

Superior doctors prevent disease.
Mediocre doctors treat the disease before the event.
Inferior doctors treat the full-blown disease.

HAUG DEE: NAI-CHING
2600BC
first Chinese medical text

introduction
GOOD HEALTH AND FITNESS ARE NOT GUARANTEES FOR A HEALTHY HEART

> *My only saving grace was that I was incredibly fortunate to find out through testing rather than my family finding out through an autopsy.*
>
> **DAN**

> *I had the sensation of both my arms feeling progressively cold and deadened from the shoulders down. I wondered, somewhat disassociated from what was happening, if this was the feeling of dying.*
>
> **RON**

> *And then, the tests come back, and they say, "You've had a heart attack, and you've got blockages in three coronary arteries. ... you're gonna have triple bypass surgery..." – and a week later, I was home. It was just a surreal experience.*
>
> **DARREN**

PATIENT'S PERSPECTIVE – DAN

I'm still unsure when I started suffering from coronary artery disease[1]. Even with the benefit of hindsight, there are no light bulb moments or signs I missed that should have warned me to take preventative action earlier than I did. No chest pain or shortness of breath that could not be excused for sickness, loss of fitness or stress.

Perhaps that's why I had no fears ahead of a trip to the doctor in mid-November 2021. It was my first visit to a GP in about three years, the previous having been for a medical that was required as part of the entry conditions to run the Paris Marathon. What started as an appointment for an ear blockage resulted in a recommendation for a complete general medical from which blood tests revealed a cholesterol level of 7.9 and my doctor's recommendation to see a cardiologist. At the time, I was not at my fittest following a stressful year at work due to COVID lockdowns and a struggling Tasmanian tourism industry. Also, a minor sporting injury had kept me from running for about eight weeks. Still, I was in reasonable shape and the last thing that crossed my mind was the potential for an issue with heart disease.

The cardiologist was reassuring. With general good health and no family history of heart disease, I don't believe either of us was overly alarmed. Still, we discussed the merits and risks of further testing, including a CT[2] heart scan used to highlight coronary artery disease. I thought that completing such a test would show a clear picture of good health. Then, perhaps with a slight diet change to reduce cholesterol, I could go on my merry way and maybe even avoid the standard cholesterol medication often prescribed for cholesterol levels as high as mine.

As a result of why I visited the doctor in the first place, I was unfortunate to need immediate ear surgery, which was performed in Sydney. The operation was successful but required a six-to-eight-week recovery period. With Christmas approaching, my scan was booked for early January, with a course of statins and aspirin prescribed as a precautionary measure.

Whilst recovering from ear surgery, I picked up a mild ear infection, which left me fatigued and, for the first time in memory, I felt short of breath following even light exercise. Nothing unexpected, I thought, given recent medications and the infection.

I remember meeting on New Year's Eve with a few from my regular running group for a 12km slow jog on the flat, a distance about half of what I had been running regularly for the past 10 years. Four kilometres in I required a 'toilet stop' just to catch my breath. Somehow, I managed to grind out the remaining eight kilometres. However, it did me no favours. I was sore for days, pulling up worse than after a marathon. Again, I put it down to the ear surgery and infection and 12 weeks of reduced exercise. I still wasn't the least bit alarmed.

I spent the first 10 days of the new year on the Tasmanian East Coast. Cleared to enter the water, I recall I struggled for breath while heading out in a large swell. That night over dinner, I discussed this with a friend's mother, a retired cardiac and ICU nurse. She told me to take these signs seriously and to get them investigated. The timing was less than a week before my scan, and it was the first time that I thought there could be more at play than a loss of fitness and a slow recovery from ear surgery. I wasn't scared, but my mind was starting to wonder.

Two days later, I had a morning run with my wife, Katie. The first kilometre was up a moderate hill – and I had to stop after 800m for a walk, something very foreign to me. Pushing on, she showed alarm at my loss of fitness and thought my ear infection and lack of exercise had taken a toll. Heart disease, however, was the furthest thing from her mind as she started plotting a diet and fitness program for me to undertake in haste.

I arrived for the scan on a Wednesday without any nerves and completed the testing without incident. However, I was surprised when I received a call from the cardiologist's office that afternoon to book a follow-up consultation that Friday for a heart stress test. I contacted my brother, who had also had a scan a few days before (ironically, he only booked after I found out about my high cholesterol). He had received no follow-up contact. Quite suddenly, a feeling of alarm came over me; I knew I wouldn't be going back for a chat about the weather.

I had had a stress test in 2012 for an insurance medical. I had completed the test (exercising on a treadmill), including three minutes at level seven, with no apparent issues and no abnormality in my exercise ECG. The conclusion then was that the test represented a "low probability of critical fixed stenosis affecting a major artery or territory". This time, the doctor aborted the test a few minutes in, and with my heart rate not exceeding 140 (far below my maximum heart rate), I knew I was in for bad news.

The tests showed that I had coronary heart disease (CHD), most likely at an advanced stage. The cardiologist recommended an invasive angiogram[3]. Whilst the angiogram can have its own risks, it was quite clear that my situation was well beyond control and such a procedure was necessary.

Suddenly, it was real, and it was significant. The angiogram was arranged for the following Wednesday. I was to have days of absolute calm in preparation for a procedure likely to change my life.

Google was my friend and foe over those days. I 'realised' (completely incorrectly) that I would need a stent, a few tablets, and a real improvement in my diet before I resumed normal life.

The day before my angiogram, I discovered that my health insurance didn't cover heart issues. Calvary Hospital, a private Hobart hospital where the angiogram was to take place, had an estimated $7000 cost for the angiogram, or I could get a booking for the Royal Hobart Hospital (RHH, 'the Royal') for the same procedure without cost. Even with expediting this due to my scan results, it would be a one-to-two-week delay.

In consideration of this, and understanding that $7000 is not an insignificant sum, I was planning to opt for the RHH option before I decided to contact a close friend who is a vascular surgeon. As luck would have it, she was with a heart surgeon at the time of the call, and as they had access to my scan, they reviewed it on the spot. I recall vividly the way she promptly stated that, in her opinion, waiting was not an option. I was worth more than $7000, and the time for waiting was over.

The angiogram itself was quite painless, and the results came back quickly. My worst fears were realised. Not only did I have coronary artery disease (CAD), but it was severe, with 95 per cent blockages consistently throughout my arteries; severe enough that I was a prime candidate for a heart attack and not an insignificant one.

My only saving grace was that I was incredibly fortunate to find out through testing rather than my family finding out through an autopsy. Whilst many CADSs are treated with stents and/or medication, I was far beyond this, and my only option was coronary artery bypass grafting (CABG).

Dan continues the very graphic account of his journey in chapter 15. Thanks to the proactive actions of his medical advisors and the modern diagnostic technology available, Dan did not suffer a heart attack. However, the consequences of his CAD were severe.

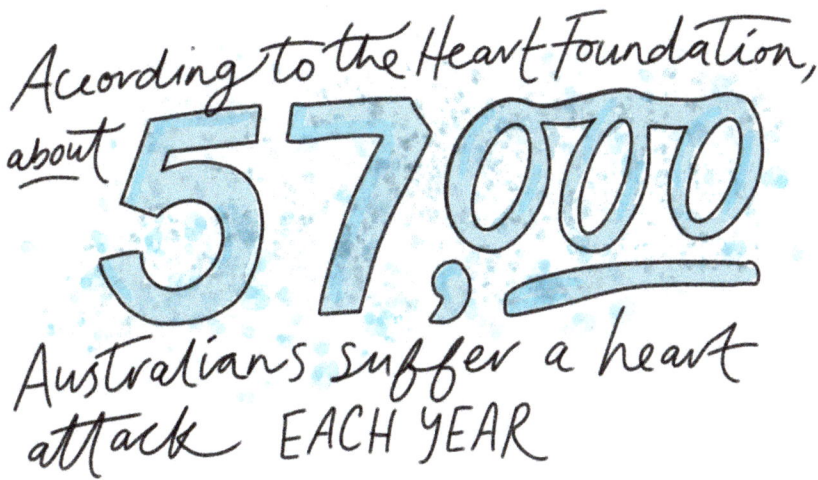

According to the Heart Foundation, about 57,000 Australians suffer a heart attack EACH YEAR

PATIENT'S PERSPECTIVE – RON

In 2018, aged 66, I was living what seemed a healthy enough life[4]. At 180cm tall, I weighed around 78kg. I didn't smoke, wasn't diabetic, mainly ate vegetarian, drank a bottle of wine over two days on the weekend and had no alcohol on the remaining five days. I rarely ate junk food and consistently observed the 5/2 fast diet, having done so for three years. At least three days a week, I walked for an hour or more. Despite this, my annual GP blood tests showed that my total cholesterol persistently hovered over 6. My GP reassured me that, despite this, given the other circumstances of my life, I needn't worry.

On a Monday morning in August 2018, I had a heart attack. I was eating breakfast when a dull ache commenced in my chest and progressively became a more painful crushing sensation. The pain was a strong pressure pain, not sharp or stabbing and, at first, not too agonising. It took a few minutes for me to start worrying that this was more than a severe bout of indigestion and possibly could be a heart attack. So, I fired up the computer and consulted 'Dr Google' – as you do these days – which reinforced my suspicion of a heart attack.

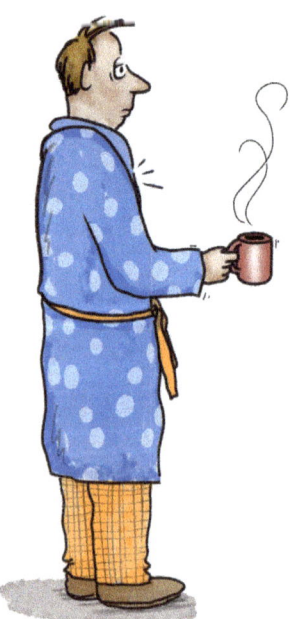

As an unfortunate result of the influence of news reports in the previous few days that ambulance ramping at the Royal Hobart Hospital meant that ambulances were delayed in responding to calls, I phoned for a taxi.

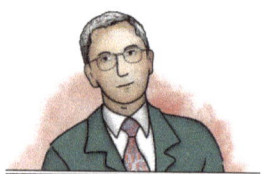

While this is Ron's retelling of his experience, the recommended response is to call 000 immediately.

During the taxi ride to the hospital, I had the sensation of both my arms feeling progressively cold and deadened from the shoulders down. I wondered, somewhat disassociated from what was happening, if this was the feeling of dying.

When I arrived at the Emergency Department, the swift response belied the frequent news reports of long waits in the ED. First, I was placed on a gurney, surrounded by medical staff, given some medication to swallow and fitted with various apparatuses. Then, while constantly being asked to rate my chest pain from one to 10, I was wheeled to another floor where I was taken for an invasive angiogram. Projecting onto a TV screen, I could see the resulting grey spidery images of blockages and near blockages in several arteries as the cardiologist explained what they were. One artery was quite blocked, and near-blockages showed in three others.

Then, I was taken to the cardiac ward and hooked up to heart monitors. I was given blood thinning medications, other medications and painkillers, and regularly asked to rate my pain from one to 10. To be honest, I found it difficult to judge how to give the pain a rating. Suffice it to say, the pain was subsiding from how it was when I first arrived at emergency, although it took about 24 hours to retreat to almost nothing.

The next few days were comfortable enough. The pain was minimal, and, it seemed a little unreal to find myself in the situation. I underwent various tests, including a CT scan and an ultrasound of my heart which identified damage to the muscle of my heart, although less damage than the medical staff had anticipated. The team of cardiologists and surgeons considered the treatments – the use of stents or coronary artery bypass surgery (CABG). Surgery was preferred because of the number of blocked or imminently blocked arteries. However, it was delayed a few days due to the amount of anti-coagulant medication I had received and the subsequent risk of bleeding.

Ron continues his gripping narrative in chapter 15.

PATIENT'S PERSPECTIVE – DARREN

I'm 50 years old[5], and on my 50th birthday, I had a heart attack[6].

I played cricket all my life[7] – 30-odd years I've been involved in cricket. I played for 20 and then have been coaching for the past 10 years with various teams. So, cricket has been my life, but suddenly, things change, you know. On February 5 (2020), at 4:30 in the morning, I woke up with cold sweats, and something's really heavy on my chest.

Oh, God!

I always was a smoker and quite a heavy smoker. And I thought, Well, I'll go have a cigarette and see if it makes it feel any better. And I didn't have the cigarette, and I went, Wow, if I don't want a cigarette, I must be in some sort of trouble.

So, I rang the doctor[8], and they got the ambulance straight around. And they gave me a spray called GTN (glyceryl trinitrate[9]) ... They gave me a spray the first time and it sort of eased off a little bit of the chest pain ... And they waited five minutes and gave me another. The paramedics were fantastic ... And then they gave me a third spray, and I felt really good. And I said, Thanks very much, lads. Off you go. Don't worry about it. And they said, No, no. You're coming with us. You're in a bad way.

And I went, Well, I feel good. What's wrong? I'm a 50-year-old. I can't be having a heart attack. This is ridiculous.

Anyway, I agreed to go with the 'ambos', and, you know, an hour later, I was in Gold Coast public hospital[10] and getting an invasive angiogram done. And then, the tests come back, and they say, You've had a heart attack, and you've got blockages in three coronary arteries. We're going to actually open you up, and you're gonna have triple bypass surgery.

After the diagnosis, Darren was moved to The Prince Charles Hospital[11] in Chermside, Brisbane, and operated on within a couple of days by cardio-thoracic surgeon Dr Peter Tesar and his open-heart surgery team.

... and a week later, I was home. It was just a surreal experience, not really understanding but trusting what the doctors were saying. I'm just so thankful that I did.

Darren explained that looking back there might have been a warning sign or two. Before the heart attack, he would have a 30-40-minute nap after training or other physical activities.

I walk or bike every day, and I still do that now, but now I can breathe. It's just amazing that you don't know. And then you get these new arteries in your heart, and you can breathe again. That was the big change.

We live in quite a hilly suburb in Brisbane. I'd go walking and by the end of it I was really short of breath. Tired and, you know, couldn't keep going. But now it's fantastic. I go up these hills, and yeah, my heart rate gets up there, but I'm up and down and I keep going. I stop when I want to stop now, not because I have to stop.

The full text of this interview features in Dr Bishop's book, *Cardiac Rehabilitation Explained* (2023) or can be accessed as podcast 161 on the **Healthy Heart Network,** https://drwarrickbishop.com/s/darren

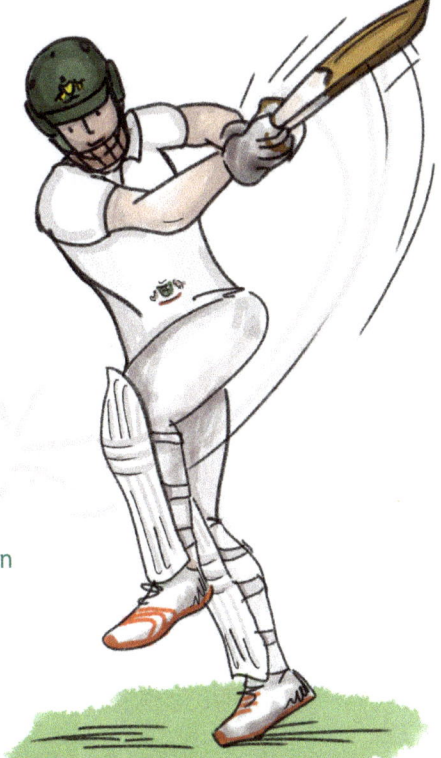

statistics don't lie

According to the (Australia) Heart Foundation[12], **more than 57,000 Australians suffer heart attacks each year**. This rate equates to **157 people being hospitalised due to a heart attack every day** or **one person every nine minutes**. Most admissions are male. While hospitalisations for heart attacks have decreased over the past 10 years, $680 million is spent annually on healthcare services related to heart attack hospitalisations, with this expenditure rising on average 3.6 per cent annually.

One person in Australia dies from a heart attack every 74 minutes or, on average, 19 people a day. Many are men and 20 per cent of them are younger than 65 years old.

'Heart attack' is a layman's term for the sudden blockage of a coronary artery that supplies oxygen-rich blood to the heart muscle. Typically, this results in the death of part of the heart muscle. The consequence **can** be fatal.

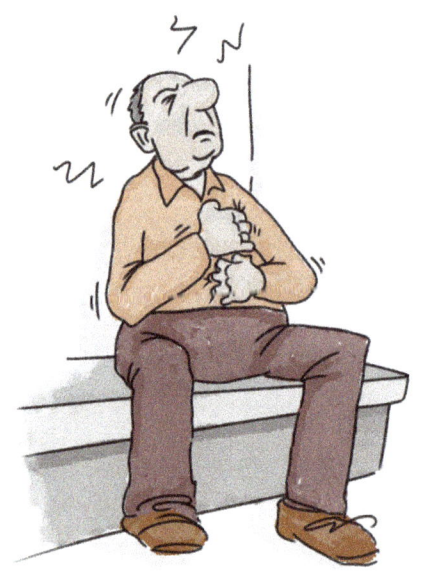

Those who survive require medical intervention – lots of medication, time in hospital, stent implantation or coronary artery bypass grafting – rehabilitation, and ongoing lifestyle modifications.

According to a World Health Organization fact sheet, 11 June 2021[13], an estimated 17.9 million people died from cardiovascular disease worldwide in 2019, representing 32 per cent of all global deaths. Of these deaths, 85 per cent were from heart attack and stroke.

For other sobering statistics from the Heart Foundation and the World Health Organization, see appendix 2, page 200.

IMPORTANT POINTS

GOOD HEALTH AND FITNESS ARE NOT GUARANTEES

- Heart attacks happen unexpectedly.
- A heart attack can kill.
- Those who survive require:
  - medical intervention, including medications, implantation of stent/s or bypass surgery
  - rehabilitation and
  - lifestyle modification.
- Although people do not plan to have one, most heart attacks are preventable.

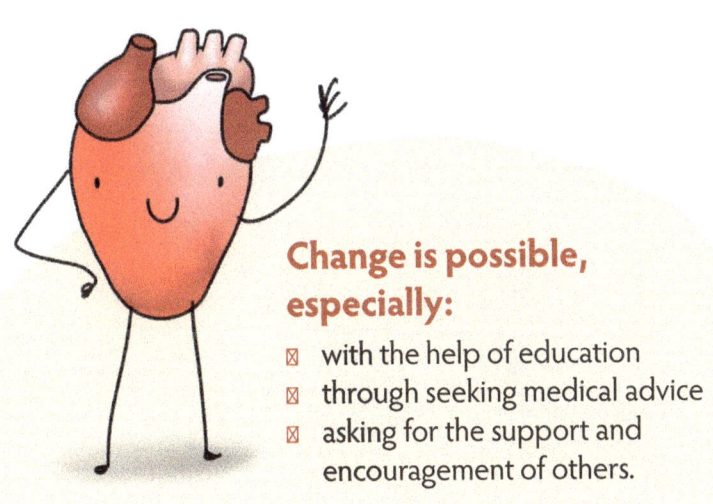

Change is possible, especially:

- ☒ with the help of education
- ☒ through seeking medical advice
- ☒ asking for the support and encouragement of others.

1. Written by Dan, 45 at the time, who lives in Hobart (Tasmania, Australia) and is a patient of Dr Bishop.
2. CT computed tomography. Current technology accurately and reliably acquires images of the arteries of the heart for evaluation of calcification. The exquisite detail gives information about the location of plaque, the quality and nature of the plaque, degree of stenosis and size of the vessel affected. Coronary computed tomography angiogram (CTCA) is often referred to as a CT coronary angiogram. (see page 147-149 for further detail)
3. This is a medical procedure in which contrast (dye) is injected into a patient to outline the coronary arteries. There are two: the non-invasive CT coronary angiogram, and the 'invasive' procedure in which the dye is injected directly into the arteries through a small tube past in through the arm or leg to the heart.
4. Written by Ron who lives in Hobart and is a patient of Dr Bishop.
5. 2020
6. From an interview between Darren Lehmann and Warrick Bishop, recorded in 2020.
7. Darren is a 27-times capped Australian Test cricketer, One Day International star, World Cup winner and top-flight Australian, state and franchise coach.
8. Darren was staying in a hotel on Queensland's Gold Coast at the time.
9. used to treat chest pain (angina)
10. Gold Coast University Hospital, Southport, Queensland
11. The Prince Charles Hospital, at Chermside, is one of the leading cardiothoracic hospitals in Australia.
12. These statistics are from the Heart Foundation website: https://www.heartfoundation.org.au/activities-finding-or-opinion/key-statistics-heart-attack
13. World Health Organization fact sheet, 11 June 2021, https://www.who.int/news-room/fact-sheets/detail/cardiovascular-diseases-(cvds)

Let's learn more about what it is that we are trying to keep healthy.

A HEALTHY HEART

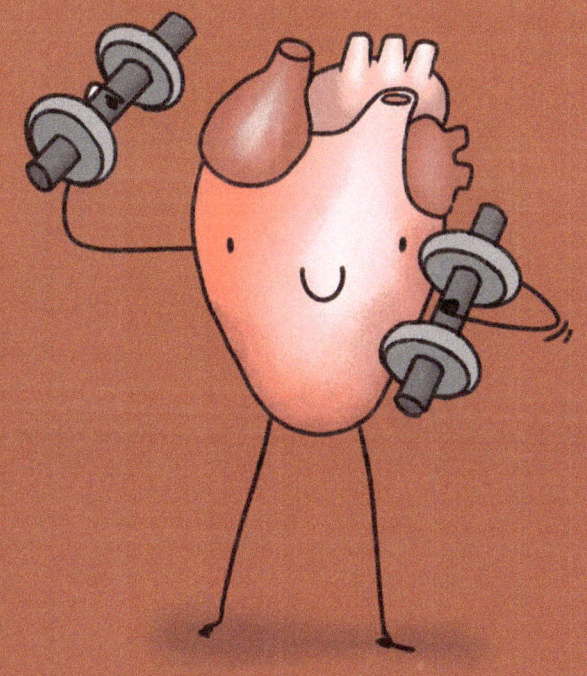

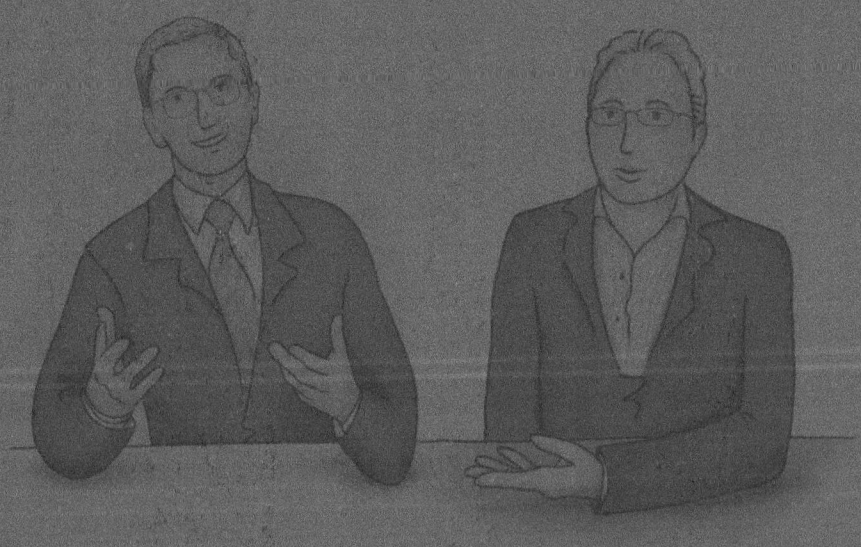

chapter 1
THE HEALTHY HEART

The heart is a large muscle that pumps blood through our bodies so that nutrients and oxygen can reach all parts of the body, and waste, such as carbon dioxide, is removed. A well-functioning heart contracts rhythmically, pumping blood to the body roughly 100,000 times a day.

Within the heart structure, there are two chambers on the right-hand side and two chambers on the left-hand side so that, on each side of the heart, there is a pre-pumping chamber, the atrium, and the main pumping chamber, the ventricle.

This means that the heart has **two pumps**, one which **accepts** the blood back from the body and then pumps it to the lungs for the carbon dioxide/oxygen exchange, and a second pump which receives the blood from the lungs and then **drives** it around the body. These are the 'right heart' and the 'left heart', respectively. The sides pump together, with each atrium contracting marginally ahead of its ventricle.

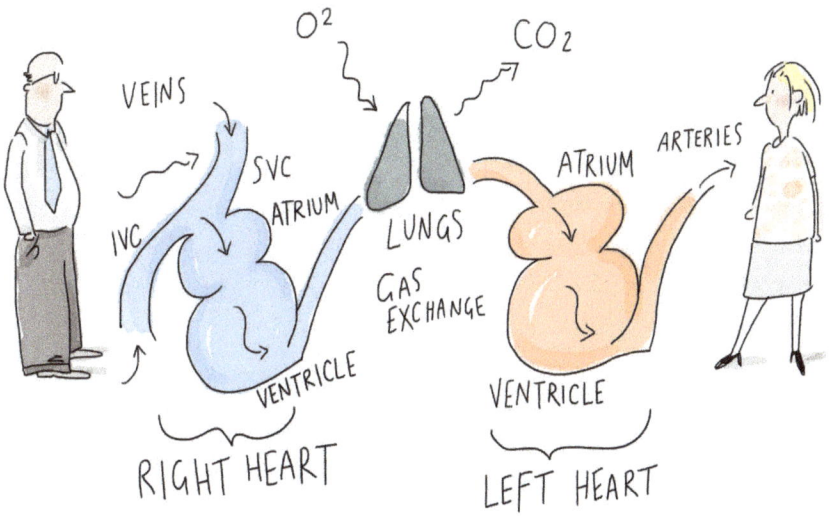

a schematic showing the flow of the blood from the veins through the heart to the arteries

The heart has three main 'systems':

- an **electrical system** for timing, which ensures synchronicity and coordinated contraction throughout the heart. It also allows for acceleration and deceleration of the heart as a pump;
- a **pumping system,** the compression chambers, the main one being the left ventricle, and several valves that stop the blood flowing back from where it has come;
- a **fuel system**, the arteries, which carries the life-blood, initially, to the heart itself (the coronary arteries) and then to the body.

the electrical system

A healthy heart is a highly efficient pump coordinated by its electrical system. The atria and ventricles work together, alternately contracting and relaxing, to pump blood through the heart and into the body. Electrical impulses trigger the heartbeat. Typically, the heart's natural pacemaker – a small area of the heart called the **sinoatrial** (SA) **node**, located at the top of the right atrium – sets off the contractions of the atria. The SA node is where the electrical activity 'beats the drum' to which the rest of the heart 'marches'.

Electrical impulses travel rapidly through the atria, somewhat like a Mexican wave, causing the muscle fibres to contract, squeezing blood into the ventricles.

To reach the ventricles, these electrical impulses pass through the **atrioventricular** (AV) **node**, a cluster of cells in the centre of the heart between the atria and the ventricles. This node acts as a gatekeeper. Passing through this node **slows** the electrical impulses before they enter the ventricles, thus giving the atria time to contract before the ventricles contract.

Once in the ventricles, specialised cells called **Purkinje Fibres** carry the electrical impulse. These fibres act like wires delivering the signal to the apex of the heart, ensuring the blood is expelled from the furthest point first.

This normal heart rhythm is known as **sinus rhythm** because the sino-atrial, or sinus, node controls it. In a healthy heart, this beating is synchronistic and smooth. Visualise, if you can, a squid moving through the water. Synchronous. Coordinated. Smooth.

When this synchronicity breaks down, heart **arrhythmias** occur. Heart arrhythmias are atrial fibrillation, atrial or ventricular ectopic beats, atrial flutter, supraventricular tachycardia, ventricular tachycardia, and ventricular fibrillation.

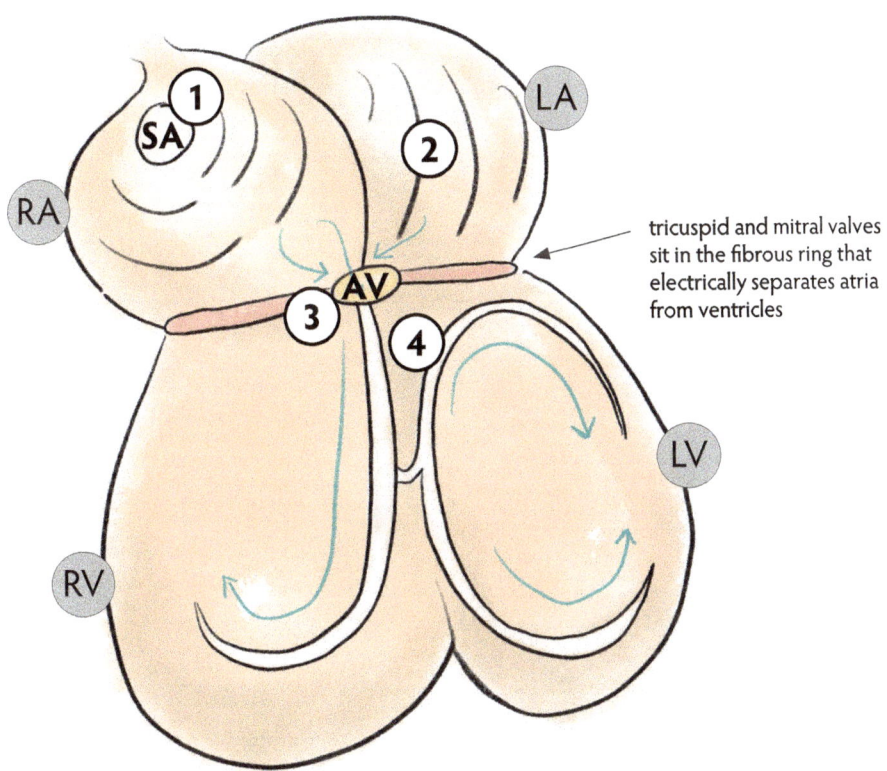

1. electrical impulse originates in SA (sinoatrial) node
2. impulse propagates through atria
3. impulse passes through AV (atrioventricular) node
4. impulse is 'delivered' to ventricles through Purkinje fibres (similar to copper wires in the heart)

the heart's 'electrical system' that coordinates a highly effective pump

the pumping system

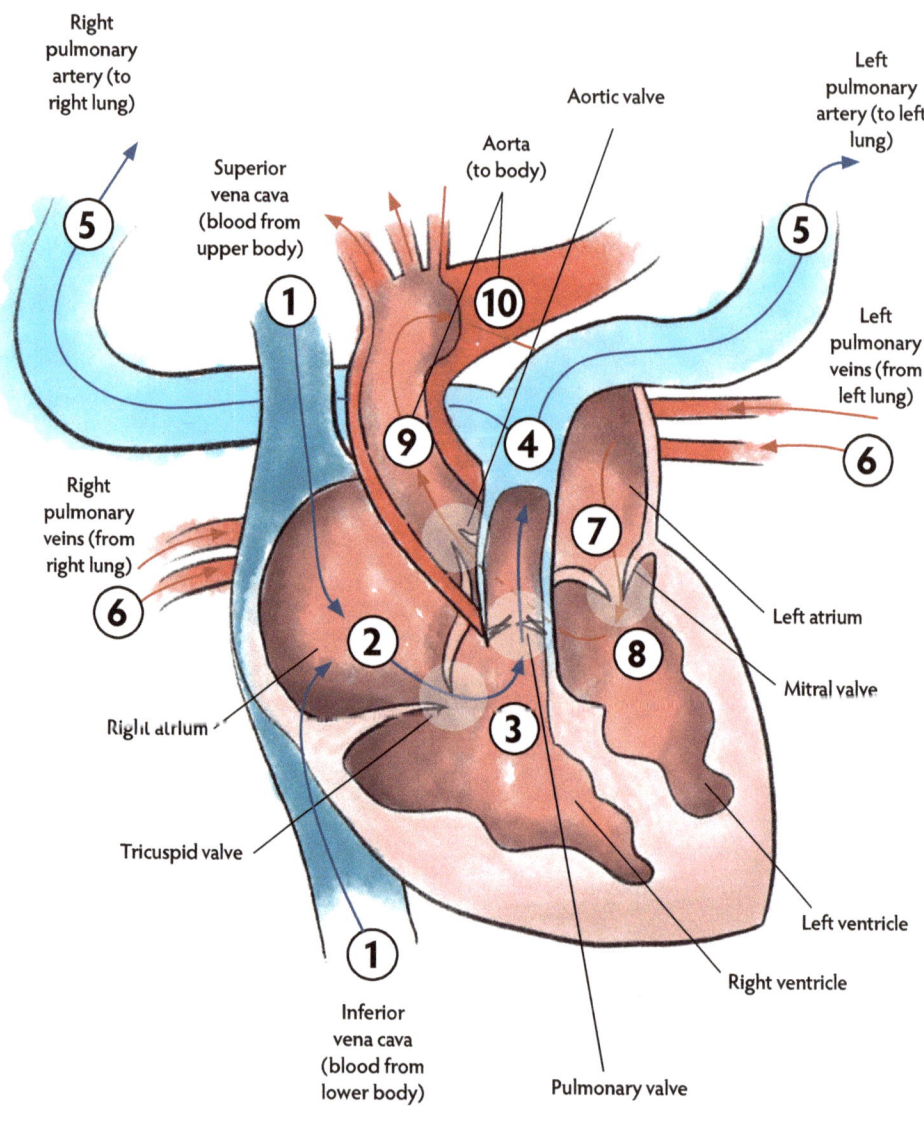

the 'pumping system', showing blood flow and connections inside the heart

The heart's pumping chambers are the **two atria** and the **two ventricles**. The **main pump is the left ventricle**.

The heart has four one-way valves – the **tricuspid**, the **pulmonary**, the **mitral**, and the **aortic** valves – that keep the blood flowing in the right direction.

Blood flows from the body to the heart through the veins, collecting into two major veins called the **superior vena cava** (SVC) ① (*refer to the diagram on the facing page*) and the **inferior vena cava** (IVC), which drain into the right side of the heart.

This oxygen-poor, dark purple, carbon dioxide-rich blood arrives in the **right atrium** ② where it receives a gentle pump through the **tricuspid valve**, a one-way valve, into the **right ventricle** ③.

The ventricle then pumps the blood through another one-way valve, the **pulmonary valve**, into the **lungs** via the **pulmonary arteries** ④, ⑤.

Within the lungs, gas exchange occurs; the air we breathe in provides oxygen, and the breath we exhale carries away carbon dioxide. As a result, the blood becomes replenished with fresh oxygen for use by the body.

Bright red, oxygen-rich arterial blood then flows from the lungs through the **four pulmonary veins** ⑥ to the **left atrium** ⑦.

The left atrium gives a gentle pump and the blood passes through the **mitral valve**, another one-way valve, into the **left ventricle** ⑧.

The left ventricle then contracts, squeezing blood through the **aortic valve**, another one-way valve, into the body's main artery, the **aorta** ⑨, ⑩, to begin its journey around the body.

the fuel system

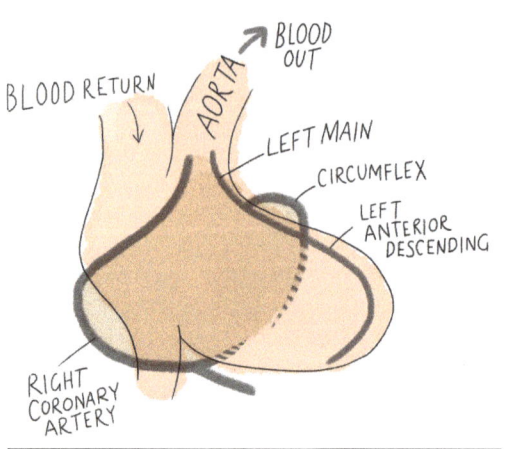

the 'fuel system', the blood vessels wrapped around the heart

As we have just seen, after the 'left' heart receives it back, the left ventricle then pumps the blood through the aortic valve into the aorta, the largest artery in the body. Almost immediately, other major arteries – the coronary arteries – branch off the aorta. This system consists of the **left main coronary artery** and the **right coronary artery**.

Within one centimetre, the **left main coronary** artery divides into two arteries:

- the **left anterior descending artery,** which provides blood to the anterior surface of the heart (the surface nearest to the chest wall), and
- the **circumflex artery,** which supplies blood to the back of the heart (the surface of the heart nearest the spine).

The **right coronary artery** supplies the inferior surface of the heart, which is the surface that is nearest the diaphragm.

The terms 'right dominant' or 'left dominant' are used in reference to the artery that supplies blood to the bulk of the inferior surface of the heart (the surface nearest the diaphragm). This blood is usually from the right coronary artery and, therefore, termed 'right dominant'. Sometimes, however, the right coronary artery is smaller, and the circumflex artery (which branches off the left main coronary artery) is bigger, or 'dominant'. Therefore, when the left coronary artery supplies most of the inferior surface of the heart, it is called 'left dominant'.

Size becomes significant in terms of the amount of the heart that may be affected by a blockage of the artery, the dominant artery providing blood to a larger territory.

Most often, the **left anterior descending artery** is the largest and most important of the three main coronary arteries. It can be 12 to 14 centimetres long while only two to five millimetres in diameter. This dimension is a little thicker than a pen refill, yet its blockage can be disastrous. A **dominant right coronary artery** can be approximately the same size, and a **non-dominant circumflex** can be six to eight centimetres long and 1.5 to three millimetres in diameter.

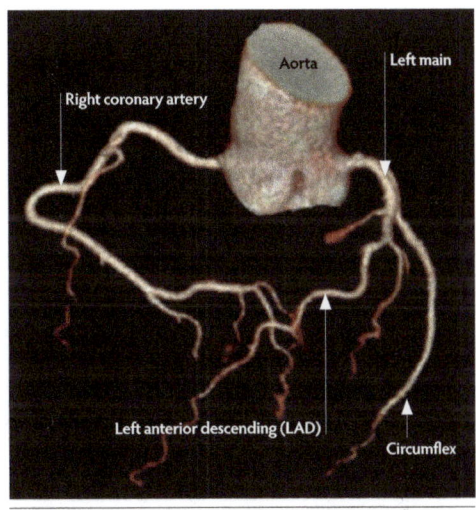

the coronary tree as seen on cardiac CT imaging

The major arteries comprise fewer than 35cm in total length and fewer than five millimetres in diameter at their largest. A single build-up of plaque leading to a blockage may only be one centimetre in length.

these coronary arteries create a very vulnerable system

left anterior descending (LAD) at actual size – the largest and most important of the coronary arteries

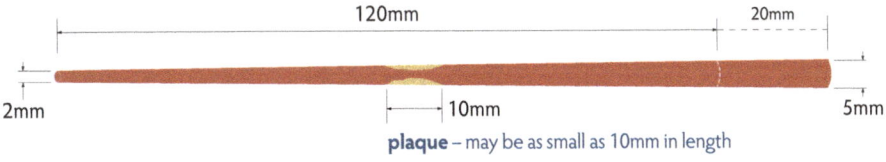

plaque – may be as small as 10mm in length

our coronary arteries create a small and vulnerable system that can be deadly

other vital components

the blood

The blood **ties the systems together**.

Blood contains **red cells** that are carriers of **haemoglobin**, the oxygen-carrying substance that transports oxygen to the body's tissues. A good supply of oxygen is critical for the proper functioning of the heart and other body organs.

Platelets are another essential component of the blood. Platelets **stop us from bleeding**, for example, when we cut ourselves. Damage within the vascular system needs these tiny particles along with fibrin to help form a thrombus (clot) and prevent the escape of blood from the body.

The blood also carries **nutrients** and **fats** such as cholesterol.

the circulation

Finally, the circulatory system **transports** the blood to the body. Keeping in mind the already-discussed sections of the heart, imagine the circulation as a closed loop like the inner tube of a tyre containing fluid that passes around the tube in one direction.

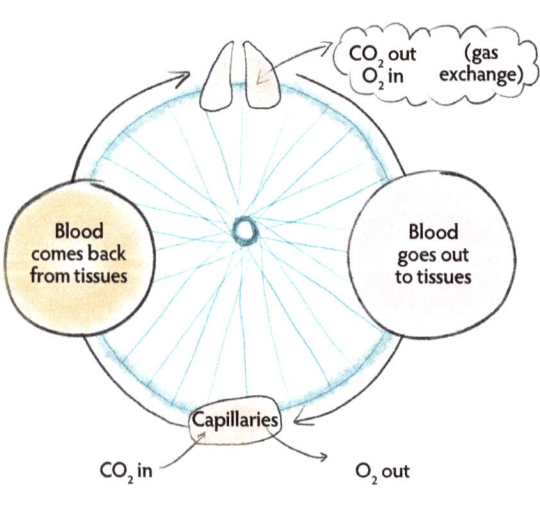

gas exchanges

Moving clockwise from the lungs at 12 o'clock, the fluid, the oxygenated blood, passes through the heart's left atrium and the left ventricle, then goes into the body to the organs, where it provides oxygen and nutrients to the tissues.

After the heart, the next major organ supplied by blood is the **brain**. Nearly 25 per cent of the blood circulating through the body goes to the brain, supplied by the carotid and the vertebral arteries. The **kidneys** need almost 25 per cent as they busily clean the blood, filtering out impurities and making urine. The **gut** gets blood; the amount varies depending on circumstances such as if you have recently had a meal. **Muscles** also receive blood, the amount of which depends on circumstances such as if you are resting or exercising.

These organs take the blood through smaller and smaller arteries, called **arterioles**, until they become very small and very fine blood vessels, the **capillaries**. They are so fine that they allow the **exchange** of oxygen and carbon dioxide through their membranes. As the blood continues its journey, the capillaries form **veins** and the veins form the IVC, which drains the lower section of the body, or the SVC, which drains the top of the body. Next, the blood passes into the right atrium and the right ventricle and circulates back into the lungs, and the cycle repeats itself.

breathing

As the lungs and the heart are within the thorax (chest cavity), breathing also impacts the return of blood through the veins (venous return). Every breath in lowers the pressure within the chest, which means that the blood outside the chest is drawn into the chest.

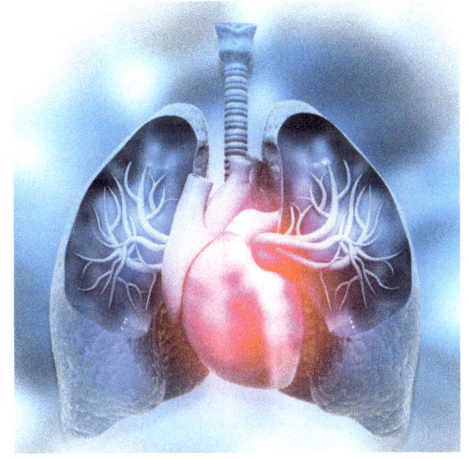

the lungs in relation to the heart

muscles

A significant amount of blood returns to the right atrium and the lungs via veins located between the muscles. These veins also have one-way valves to ensure the blood continues to flow in a clockwise direction as it is 'pumped' by the contraction of the nearby muscle.

IMPORTANT POINTS

THE HEALTHY HEART

- The heart is a muscle that pumps blood around the body
  - taking oxygen-rich blood from the lungs to the organs, tissues, and muscles, and
  - returning oxygen-depleted/carbon dioxide-rich blood to the lungs where an oxygen-carbon dioxide exchange occurs.
- The heart has three main systems:
  - an electrical system that ensures synchronicity, co-ordination, and rate;
  - a pumping system with compression chambers and valves, and
  - a fuel system, the coronary arteries, that takes the blood from the heart chambers to the heart muscle, the beginning of the journey of the blood around the body.

Let's now turn our attention to understanding a heart attack.

chapter 2
HOW DOES A HEART ATTACK HAPPEN?

The heart – the large muscle that pumps blood through our bodies – is the crucial organ for sustaining life in the human body.

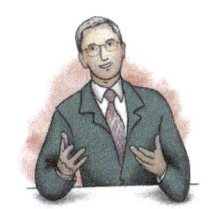

Critical to the heart's operations are three major arteries, the coronary arteries. These fuel lines carry oxygen-rich blood to the heart muscle so that it can contract rhythmically, pumping blood to the body 35 million times a year to deliver nutrients and oxygen and remove waste such as carbon dioxide.

The heart pumps three to four litres of blood every minute, with a healthy heart rate of between 50 and 100 beats per minute.

why do we care?

Heart attack is a big deal[14]:

heart attack statistics	
1 in 4 deaths	Western World
1 death every 40 seconds	United States of America
1 death every 74 minutes	Australia
1 in 5 deaths	65 years or less

ANSWERING YOUR QUESTIONS

what does a healthy artery look like?

A healthy artery (*see diagram, right*) consists of an inner layer of endothelial cells (*pictured top in the diagram*), a middle layer of smooth, muscle cells (*middle*), and an outer layer of collagen (*bottom*).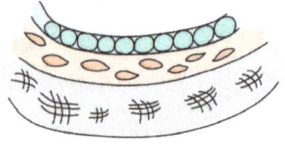

The inner layer **(tunica intima – meaning inner coat)** is a smooth lining made from sheets of cells called the endothelium (endo, inside; thelium, skin). This unique layer of cells ensures the blood's contents run smoothly through a blood vessel and do not stick or clump to the side walls. As well as acting as a 'Teflon lining', the endothelium also responds to stressors and strain within the artery and then communicates with the muscle layer of the artery to influence relaxation or contraction.

The middle layer **(tunica media – middle coat)** is made up predominately of muscle cells. These are special muscle cells called smooth muscle. They are different to the muscle in your leg, which is skeletal muscle (or, in your heart, for that matter, which is cardiac muscle). Smooth muscles are not controlled by nerves in the way the skeletal muscles are, but they respond to the automatic regulatory systems of the body. (You find smooth muscle in the wall of the stomach, gut, bladder, and ureters.) If you were to be frightened, the body's automatic (called the autonomic) nervous system would go into overdrive, pumping adrenaline into the bloodstream and activating its own special nerves, leading to stimulation of the blood vessels' smooth muscle. As the smooth muscle contracts, it narrows the artery. As the same amount of blood is being pumped through narrower blood vessels, this increases blood pressure. So, this layer of the blood vessel has a significant influence on blood pressure regulation. (WB: This is oversimplified, but it conveys the basic idea.)

The outer layer **(tunica adventitia – outside coat)**, the main scaffold of the artery, consists of collagen, the tissue that binds together almost all tissues in the body. The outer walls of the major arteries are, and must be, very tough to deal with years of pulsating blood being forced through the body. Interestingly, the stretch and recoil of the walls of those big arteries act as a secondary pump for the body, maintaining the flow between heartbeats.

The term 'heart attack' is a layman's term for what, in medicine, is called **myocardial ischemia** (myocardial, pertaining to the heart muscle; ischemia, lack of blood) or **myocardial infarction** (infarction, death from lack of blood flow). Sometimes, it is called a **major adverse coronary event** (MACE) and comes under the umbrella of **acute coronary syndrome** (acute, happens suddenly; coronary, heart arteries; syndrome, problem).

A heart attack is a significant problem caused by the sudden blocking of one or more coronary arteries resulting in reduced or no blood flow to the heart muscle.

Heart attack arises from **coronary artery disease** (CAD). On rare occasions, a heart attack can happen due to a coronary dissection (tear in the blood vessel) or even more rarely, a blood clot alone. **Angina** and **shortness of breath** are the main CAD symptoms. A heart attack requires urgent medical intervention – medication, hospitalisation, stents or coronary bypass grafting – rehabilitation and ongoing lifestyle modification.

The process leading to a heart attack begins many years before – sometimes in our teens – in an artery where plaque (a cholesterol-rich deposit) starts to build up. Think of rust in a pipe that has water constantly rushing through it. Think of arteries with blood continuously being pumped through them. Both systems are subject to general wear and tear and breakdowns in localised spots.

what is plaque?

As the previous page tells us, a **healthy artery** consists of three layers of cells, with Teflon-like endothelial cells forming the inner layer, which prevents blood components from sticking and clogging up the arteries.

If that layer becomes inflamed in a local spot – by the movement of blood generating shear stress – it sends messages that set off a chain of events that brings cholesterol into that area to begin the repair process (cell membrane construction needs cholesterol). Further messages let the body know cholesterol – the **low-density lipoprotein, LDL cholesterol**, the so-called 'bad' cholesterol – is now where it normally wouldn't be.

(continued page 45)

ANSWERING YOUR QUESTIONS

what is cholesterol?

The word cholesterol has its origins in Greek: chole (bile) and stereos (solid), followed by the chemical suffix -ol (alcohol).

Cholesterol is a waxy, fat-like, organic (found in living systems) substance that is an essential component of all animal cells. So, it is important, and there is a lot of it in the body. However, cholesterol is central to the build-up of plaque, one of the most important risk factors for heart attack/stroke and heart disease.

Several hormones need cholesterol in their making, such as the adrenal gland hormones, which include mineralocorticoids (these help control fluid balance and electrolytes in the body) and glucocorticoids (these are involved in the body's immune response). Cholesterol is also the basic building block for the sex hormones progesterone, oestrogen and testosterone and their derivatives. Cholesterol is a precursor to synthesising (or making) vitamin D in the body.

All cells in the body can make cholesterol. However, we also consume foods that contain cholesterol. The body absorbs about 50 per cent of the cholesterol it ingests. Cholesterol levels in the bloodstream vary. Genetics determine this variability such that even significant dietary efforts to alter cholesterol levels will rarely achieve greater than 15 per cent changes in the measured blood cholesterol levels – a source of great frustration to many patients!

Cholesterol is carried through the body by particular proteins, called lipoproteins. There is a fair amount of complexity to this. However, in the simplest terms, a protein carrier takes cholesterol from the liver to the tissues. This protein is called low-density lipoprotein (LDL) and is often referred to as 'bad' cholesterol. The protein that tends to carry cholesterol back to the liver is called high-density lipoprotein (HDL), the 'good' cholesterol. A balance is required: bad cholesterol puts cholesterol into the arteries, and good cholesterol takes it away. Hence, the ratio of 'bad' cholesterol to 'good' cholesterol has historically been a mainstay in assessing the likelihood of a build-up of cholesterol in the arteries which is then complicit in the formation of plaque.

(from page 43)

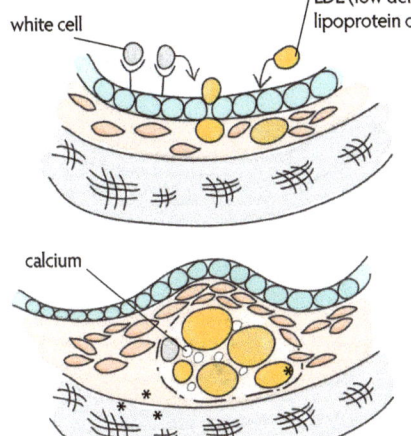

at the site of damage to endothelium
White cells and cholesterol (LDL) are drawn into the artery at the site of damage or trauma to the endothelium.

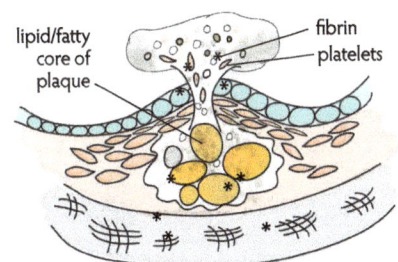

development of plaque
White cells and cholesterol collect in plaque as macrophages and lead to scarring. Calcium moves into scarred areas of plaque.

rupture of plaque and formation of clot (thrombosis)
Blood contents react with the contents of the plaque when it ruptures. A clot forms.

As cholesterol liberates chemicals within the artery's wall, white cells – **leukocytes,** our body's inflammatory (or immune) response – move in. Some of those white cells mature into cells called **macrophages** – big fat cells that gobble up stuff, in this case, the deposited and now redundant cholesterol. The trouble is they gobble up too much fatty cholesterol, become **foam cells**, and burst.

Because macrophages are the 'garbage guts' of the immune system, these foam cells have enzymes and other contents that spill when they rupture in the artery wall. Those enzymes have destructive properties and cause **local micro-scarring**, creating a **scaffold** on which **calcium** deposits. This inflammation process forms a collection of cholesterol, scarred material and calcium – **plaque** or coronary atherosclerosis.

In some people, this is all that happens. The process is benign; the repair satisfies the body's needs.

If the process is out of balance, so that injury continues, plaque build-up may progress until it narrows the artery and reduces the blood flow, or the plaque ruptures, forms a clot on the rupture and blocks the artery.

detection

Historically, the first time a problem with the arteries can be suspected is when symptoms – angina, shortness of breath or an acute coronary syndrome – present or an autopsy has been held.

angina	Angina is the term given to discomfort in the chest when pain is experienced in association with exertion. The term has its root meaning in a sense of strangulation.
shortness of breath on exertion	Shortness of breath on exertion can indicate a lack of blood flowing to the heart. Under these circumstances the heart cannot work properly, pressures within the pumping chamber begin to rise with back pressure to the lungs and, consequently, the person experiences shortness of breath.
acute coronary syndrome	An acute coronary syndrome is the sudden development of a complete, or near complete, blockage of a coronary artery. A lessened blood flow to a region of heart muscle results in damage. A complete blockage causes the death of that area of the heart muscle. A partial blockage, or 'unstable angina', puts strain on the heart and can be a forerunner to a complete blockage.

A build-up of plaque within an artery can be either **flow-limiting** or **non-flow-limiting.**

Autopsies after **sudden cardiac death** from coronary artery disease show that about 60 per cent of the plaques have been **flow-limiting**, or tight, before the event that led to death and, hence, likely to have **given a clue** by way of a symptom such as chest pain or shortness of breath on exertion.

So, about 40 per cent were **non-flow limiting**. In this situation, the person has **no warning** and no chance to seek help before the event. In this no-warning scenario, **death strikes suddenly**, often in a seemingly fit and healthy person.

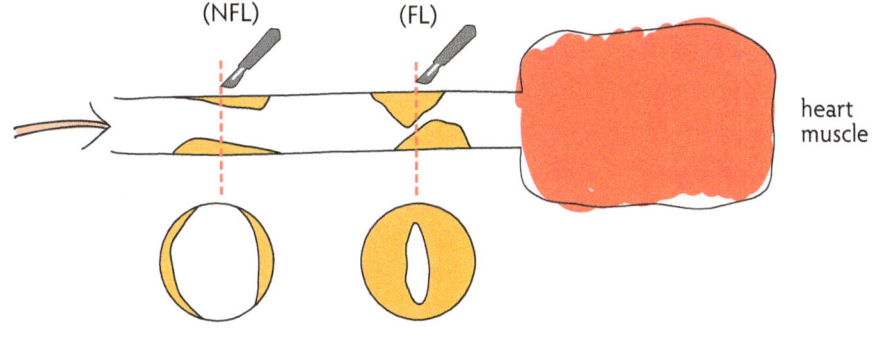

a schematic showing the components of non-flow-limiting and flow-limiting plaque are the same, just to a different extent

While flow-limiting and non-flow-limiting plaques have the same components,

- the wall of the artery
- the lumen (or inside space) of the artery
- the plaque which has built up and is beginning to intrude into the artery, and
- the fibrous cap that separates the plaque from the blood,

flow-limiting plaques are often harder and more calcified.

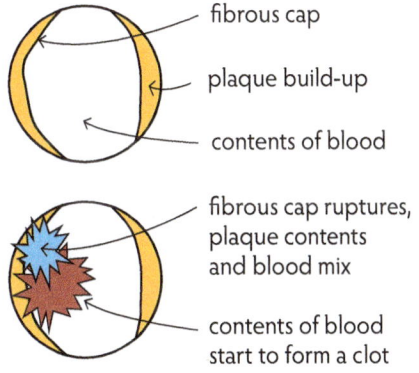

clot formation

The fibrous cap covering the plaque build-up can rupture, bringing the plaque contents into contact with the blood. Among the different components making up the blood are **platelets**, small particles central to the formation of a clot. When the blood encounters the contents of the plaque, the platelets, having detected the change, rapidly clump together with fibrin (a blood-borne protein) to form a **clot** because they think the body is under attack or bleeding.

(continued page 50)

A CLOSER LOOK

formation of a clot

The body needs to be able to protect itself if there is damage to the circulation. If unwanted bleeding is not stopped, the person will bleed to death. The mechanism that stops us bleeding to death is the formation of a blood clot, or thrombosis.

The formation of a clot needs the coagulation cascade, which has two major components. One component is the small particles that come from the bone marrow and are called **platelets.** They don't have a nucleus, so they are not 'complete' cells but they are part of what forms a clot. The other element, in conjunction with platelets, is a strong cross-bridging strand protein called **fibrin,** the scaffold of the clot formation.

When there is damage to the blood vessel, proteins and receptors that are not normally exposed to the blood circulation become exposed. With this, platelets meet receptors with which they normally would not have contact. Those proteins and receptors activate platelets, causing changes which lead to preparation for forming a clot. So that fibrin is formed to bind with those platelets, a cascade of different factors is started. That cascade is called the coagulation cascade.

The clot formation occurs through the activation of platelets which results in the platelets interacting with fibrin, after the fibrin has been generated through the coagulation cascade. Fibrin and platelets together form the clot that blocks or seals the blood vessel.

What then stops the clot progressing until all the blood congeals?

So that the whole body doesn't end up as one big clot, there are also factors generated that limit the progression of a clot. These factors are called the fibrinolytic system. As the body is forming a clot, it is also producing factors that prevent the clot from extending too far.

In some medical situations, the body does not want a clot to form as it can cause a more serious problem, such as a stroke. To help prevent a clot forming, anti-coagulation therapies are implemented, keeping in mind two major risks: the possibility of stroke in the future and the likelihood of bleeding.

A CLOSER LOOK

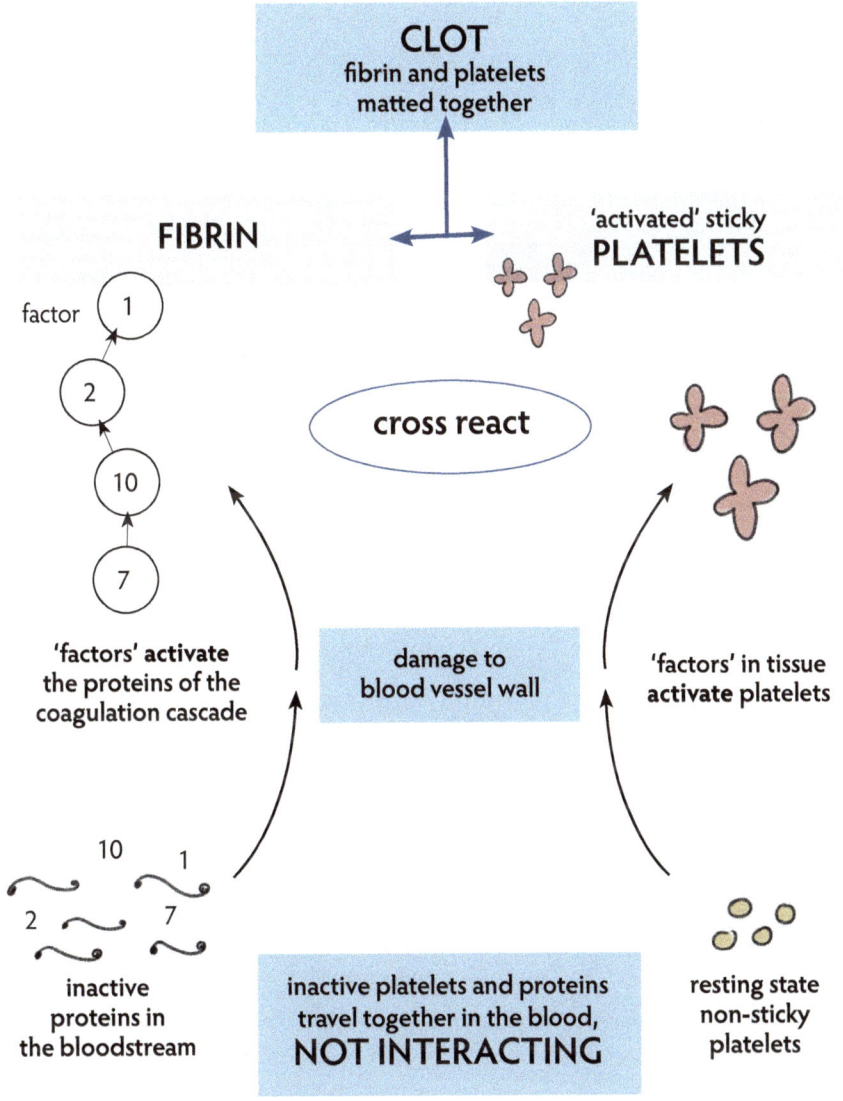

simplified schematic of the formation of a blood clot

Understanding something about the clot-forming pathway helps patients understand where and why medications work. For example, aspirin is used to dampen down platelet function. Other drugs, such as warfarin, work on different areas of the coagulation cascade, essentially to decrease the production of fibrin, and so reduce the possibility of an unwanted clot forming.

(from page 47)

Even a microscopic tear in the fibrous cap of a plaque can lead to the formation of a clot, which can then rapidly block off the artery and be life-threatening or even life-ending.

The artery, being only a couple of millimetres in width, blocks suddenly stopping the blood flow to the heart muscle. As a result, **myocardial ischaemia** – the muscle is *short* of blood – occurs; if left for too long, **myocardial infarction** – *death* of the muscle – follows. Both can be fatal.

Lack of blood impairs muscle function and so can alter the heart's electrical rhythm. If normal rhythm consequently becomes abnormal rhythm, **cardiac arrest** occurs, which **kills** the person in more than **90 per cent** of cases.

For a significant number of people – those with non-flow-limiting plaque – they feel well until the moment the artery closes off. No symptoms. No clues. No warning.

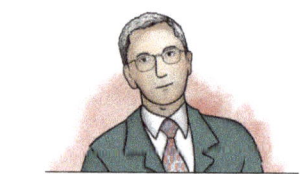

One in six people who suffer a heart attack die, and many have no warning.

A CLOSER LOOK

heart attack

Heart attack most commonly relates to a sudden blockage (due to the rupture of plaque) of one of the major arteries supplying blood to the heart muscle. Generally, it presents as chest pain, sweating, shortness of breath and, sometimes, collapse. **The person is conscious and breathing**. In this medical emergency, the patient must be taken immediately to the nearest hospital to have that artery reopened.

(sudden) cardiac arrest

Lack of blood flow to the heart muscle can lead to an electrical problem called ventricular fibrillation (ventricular, relating to the main pumping chambers of the heart; fibrillation, chaotic twitching of muscle fibres). This is a sudden cardiac arrest (SCA). The person – **collapsed, not conscious and not breathing** because the heart is not pumping – **needs immediate cardio-pulmonary resuscitation** (CPR), and, if available, use of a **defibrillator** which applies an electric 'shock' to stop the fibrillation and 'restart' the heart. Such action can be lifesaving.

Defibrillation is effective in over 90 per cent of cases if applied within one minute, but ineffective in over 90 per cent if applied 10 minutes later, even if CPR is performed.[15]

Other causes of SCA include inherited problems within the heart's electrical system or of the muscle of the heart.

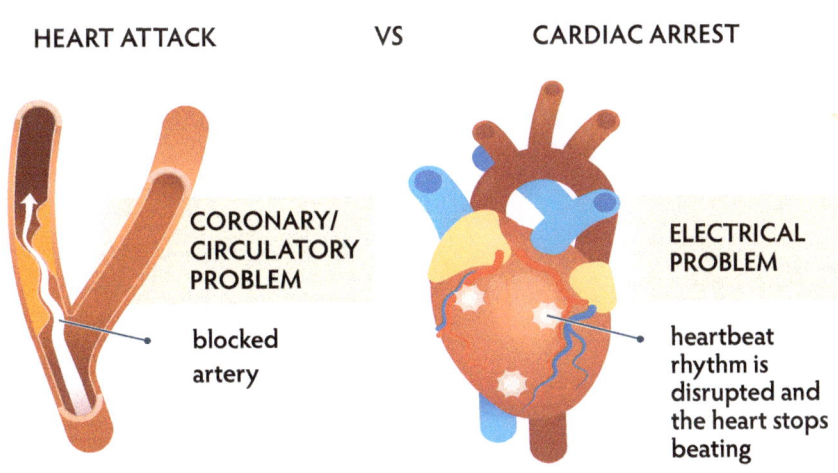

cardiac imaging

As we have already noted, for a very long time, it was not possible to look directly into the coronary arteries in a healthy person. Today, however, **cardiac imaging** plays an increasingly important role in the **early detection** and **prevention** of potential heart issues, including heart attack. As we are seeing, ascertaining the health or otherwise of the coronary arteries is so important as, in many situations, **remedial** action is available.

Cardiac health, cardiovascular prevention, well-being, knowing your risk, and dealing with any issues that arise (before or after an event) are essential to living as well as possible for as long as possible.

Occasionally, patients and even colleagues say they don't want to know what's going on with their hearts in case it is bad news. Sticking your head in the sand will not solve anything, nor allow sensible planning, whatever the situation. My response (WB) is, *Do you have your car serviced? If you do, why?*

The choice between finding out about a potential brake fault before taking the family on holiday or risking a serious or life-threatening accident is a no-brainer.

Finding out about potential problems might result in confronting information, but what's the alternative? And – you are still alive to do something about it.

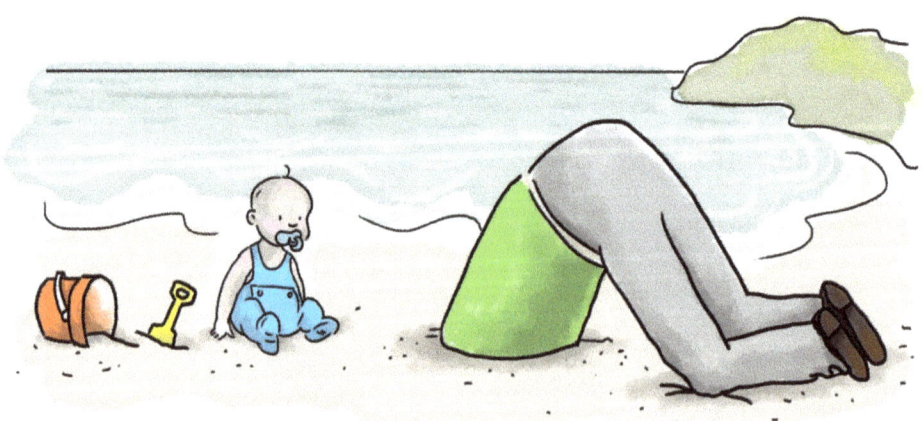

IMPORTANT POINTS

HOW DOES A HEART ATTACK HAPPEN?

- A reliable heart is essential for life.
- The death rate and distress caused by heart attacks worldwide make them the biggest health deal.
- Severely reduced or completely blocked blood flow to the heart causes a heart attack.
- Cholesterol (LDL) and white cells are drawn to localised areas of the artery when the Teflon-like inner lining, the endothelium, is damaged by wear and tear. The white cells mature into macrophages that consume cholesterol, becoming foam cells. These cells eventually burst or die, releasing enzymes that cause local scarring and, with other cellular debris, contribute to a scaffold that can become calcified.
- Plaque is the collection of cholesterol and inflammatory cells that lead to scar tissue and calcium.
- Although it starts as a process to heal the artery, it can progress to causing problems, even death.
- The plaque build-up is localised and can be flow-limiting (which generally, although not always, produces symptoms) or non-flow-limiting (which has no symptoms).
- In either case, unstable plaque can rupture, and a clot can form very quickly, blocking the artery and suddenly reducing or cutting off blood supply to the heart muscle. This can mean death of the heart muscle and, sometimes, the individual.

---

14   These figures come from the World Health Organization.
15   O'Rourke, M. F. (2010) Reality of Out of Hospital Cardiac Arrest, BMJ Journals.

Do we hope for the best or expect the worst?

chapter 3
BEING AHEAD OF THE GAME

For many years, the medical profession's approach to heart attack has been to respond after an event and has focused mainly on **secondary prevention** or dealing with risk **after** a problem has declared itself. **Symptoms** associated with a shortage of blood flowing to the heart include shortness of breath and chest pain (angina) on exertion.

On having diagnosed a patient, treatment is based on:
- understanding exactly **where** the problems are within the coronary arteries so that decisions can be made about whether re-establishing or improving blood flow with the use of stents or coronary artery bypass grafting is appropriate – **revascularisation**,
- trying to prevent another event or a further problem from occurring – **secondary prevention**.
- Strategies to reduce the risk of recurrence include:
- the **use of medication** to keep the platelets from clumping together and forming blockages in the arteries; this approach most commonly uses aspirin;
- **reducing cholesterol levels** to targets associated with significant improvement in outcome, often using cholesterol-lowering agents such as statins;
- **lifestyle modifications** that may reduce the risk: a heart-healthy diet, exercise, weight loss, blood pressure control and/or diabetes treatment, and stopping smoking.

Secondary prevention **is** beneficial in reducing the recurrence of an event as these patients have a significant build-up of cholesterol in their arteries. Secondary prevention data are unambiguous, and we (WB, KK) do not believe there is any need for alternative interpretations or strategies.

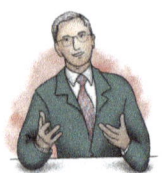

While my patients (WB) would tell you I adopt an almost boot camp mentality in my use of secondary prevention measures, from my perspective, the timing of secondary prevention is late in the process, and this presents a problem. You wouldn't want to die on your way to a secondary prevention intervention!

The situation is not so sharply defined when it involves patients who have not yet had a heart event. These people may be at high risk because of **indicators** such as cholesterol levels or blood pressure, diabetes, or even smoking, yet they do not display any symptoms, nor have they been defined as having a problem. Even so, these patients may carry an increased risk. The treatment for that risk – **before** an event – is **primary prevention,** my (WB) particular interest.

Our objective is to avoid the first event. We believe that current primary prevention practice has scope for *re-evaluating the approach to risk assessment in individuals* before they exhibit a problem. For us, preventing the chest pain and complications of a heart attack are the Holy Grail of preventative cardiology.

The difficulty with primary prevention is that it involves the **unrevealed**:

- considering a person's treatment **before** there are symptoms indicating a significant build-up of plaque within the arteries;
- deciding on the person's level of **risk**;
- the **probability** of an event occurring.

calculating risk

Observational data underpins the way that we evaluate and calculate risk in individuals. This method means that, over the years, databases have been collated of features and factors found in individuals with coronary artery disease.

The occurrence of those features and factors then lends weight to their being used as **predictors** for people **before they have an event**. This

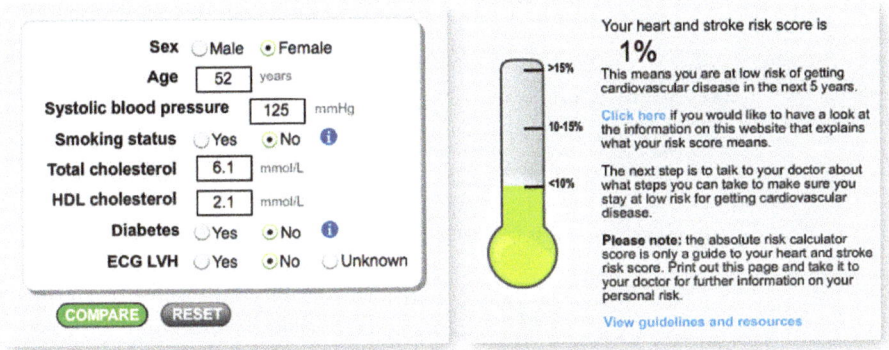

simply means that observational data collected on many patients who have had heart attacks indicate that factors such as increasing age, male sex, increased blood pressure, diabetic status and smoking all feature as **associations** to having had a coronary event.

This type of risk modelling, using **multiple associations with observed outcomes**, was first published, and used by the Framingham Group[16] in the United States of America. This Framingham-type risk modelling continues to form the basis of our current risk assessment in primary prevention[17]. Similar risk calculation tools exist in Europe and New Zealand and Australia.

understanding risk

From a cardiology perspective, we define the risk of a coronary artery event as 'low', 'intermediate', or 'high'.

- Low **risk** is considered a less than 10 per cent chance of a coronary event within 10 years.
- High **risk** is considered a greater than 20 per cent chance of an event within 10 years.
- Intermediate **risk** is between 10 and 20 per cent risk of an event within 10 years.

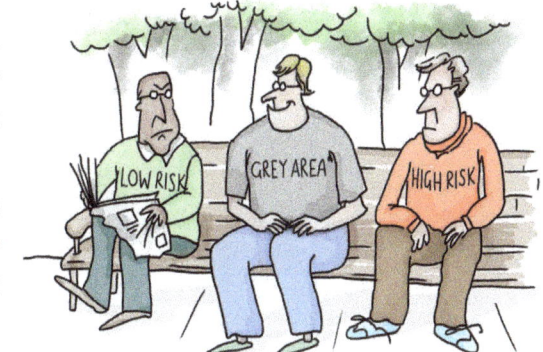

Using these risk definitions means that if we were to take a group of 100 high-risk people and follow them for 10 years, 20 or more of those people would have a coronary event.

If we introduced aspirin and a cholesterol-lowering tablet to reduce the risk of an event in this group of 100, then, statistically, *we would be treating up to 80 people who were **not** going to have an event and perhaps did **not** need treatment.*

Such a management plan would significantly impact the assessed effectiveness of that intervention. The people within the population not destined to have an event **dilute** the statistical significance of the efficacy of primary prevention in this group.

Similarly, if we were to take a group of 100 people with a low risk of an event and follow them for 10 years, up to 10 individuals could have a coronary event and 90 would remain without any symptoms or signs. Here again, the problem is: *How do we appropriately treat the 10 but not over-treat the 90?*

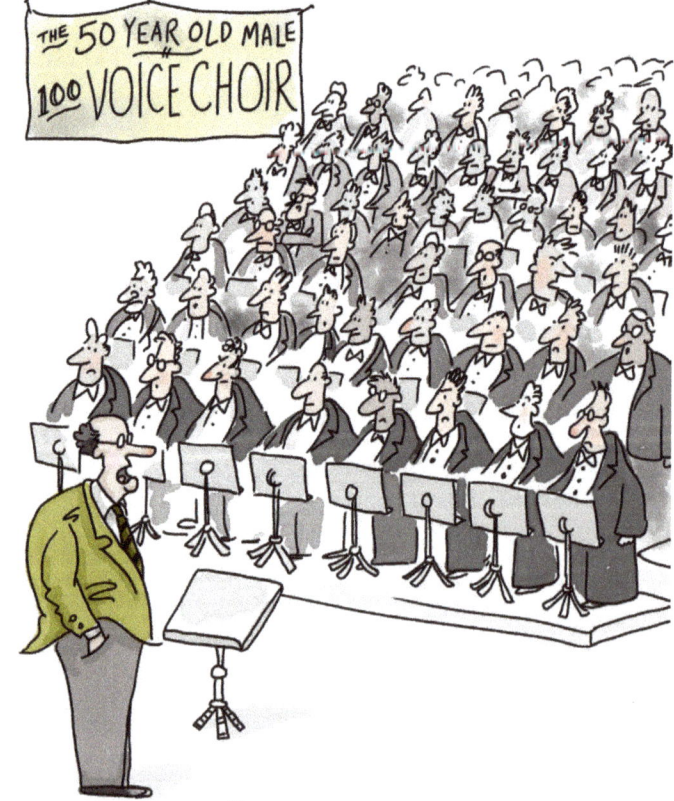

"OK guys, I've spoken to the doc and he says 10 to 15 of you will have a heart attack in the next 10 years. Could I just ask that it's not all the tenors?"

Interestingly, within the context of our medical classification, we are happy to refer to low risk as up to a 10 per cent chance within 10 years and not consider treatment, even though this could be expressed as a one per cent chance per annum of having a major event. So, how would you react if, the next time you checked in for a commercial airline flight, you were told there was a one per cent per annum chance of being involved in a crash or a 10 per cent chance of being involved in a crash over your next 10 years of flying? Unacceptable!

understanding individual risk profiles

The interesting thing is that this observational data that we have been discussing are **associations** and not necessarily **causations**, the mechanisms that cause the problem. The difference between associations and causations means that there can be people at high risk based on factors such as age, sex, and cholesterol levels who never have an event. Conversely, some people would appear to score low on these risk calculators but still have a coronary problem.

associations vs causations

Let's look at this from outside the medical field. We know that speeding and alcohol consumption are significant associations of car accidents. However, we also know that people drive over the speed limit with high alcohol levels, yet they do not have accidents. Conversely, people who drive safely can be involved in an accident. Driving within the speed limit or not consuming alcohol when driving simply **alters** the risk profile. It means that speed and alcohol are associations with having an accident. If they were causations, then every time someone sped or consumed alcohol, that person would be involved in a crash.

When it comes to the heart, I (WB) regularly need to advise patients that they have cholesterol build-up in the arteries. Often, I receive the reply:

"But Doctor, my cholesterol is fine."

"But Doc., I exercise regularly."

"But Doctor, I eat healthy food and keep my weight down."

These patients are expressing a belief that is **broadly accepted** but **universally misleading**: that certain factors, such as elevated cholesterol, lack of exercise, eating poorly or being overweight, are the **direct causes** of coronary artery disease.

They are not the *causes*; they are *associations*.

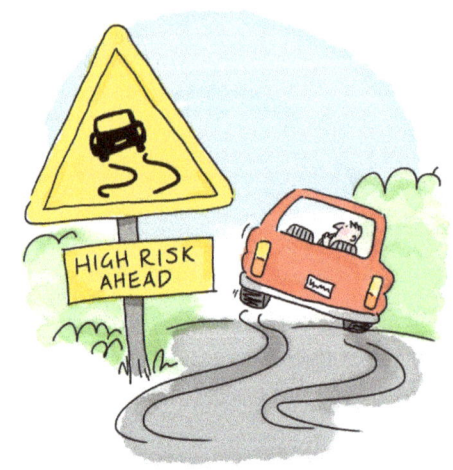

Let's go back to our car accident. Alcohol does not cause the car accident; it does not drive the car. Yet, alcohol can impair the driver's reflexes and assessment and **contribute** to that driver having an accident. The actual **cause** of the accident may be the driver approaching a sharp bend too quickly or losing concentration, a dog running out onto the street, or a car in front stopping unexpectedly.

Multiple associations can be present, yet even when put together, they do not necessarily mean that the car will be involved in an accident – just that there is **a higher risk**.

The reverse is also true. There may be no alcohol, no speeding, and an experienced driver at the wheel in good weather, yet, without any associations present, an accident occurs.

- being aware of your blood pressure and keeping it down,
- being aware of your cholesterol and dealing with it appropriately,
- undertaking regular exercise,
- not smoking, and
- addressing other cardiovascular risks

are all important for a safe journey through life. However, on their own, they offer **no guarantee** of avoiding a heart attack, although they are likely to **reduce the risk**.

We know, both from literature and personal experience,

- of people with high cholesterol levels who do not have heart attacks,
- of people who exercise regularly and have a heart attack, seemingly out of the blue at a young age,
- of people who smoke, are overweight and do not exercise, who live long lives without heart health problems, and
- of family clusters in which major adverse coronary events occur at a much higher frequency but not in all members.

the art of good medicine

The role of an experienced medical practitioner is to evaluate the individual and that person's particular needs and then, knowing and being familiar with the evidence base and the experience of other individuals, reach a conclusion that leads to an appropriate management plan.

I (WB) explain this to my patients in a way that paints a doctor a little like an astronomer.

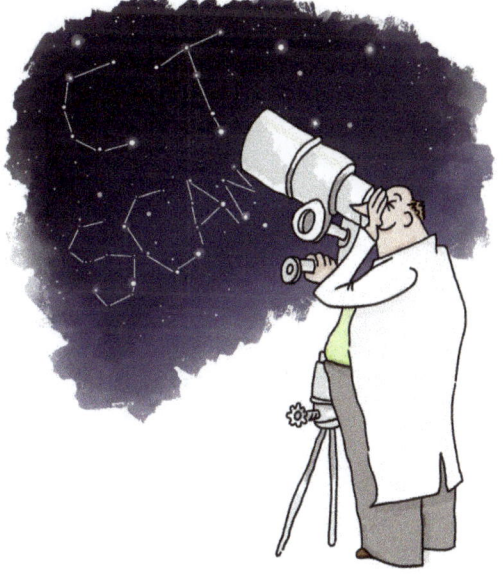

We look out into the universe that we do not fully understand, nor do we fully know its boundaries. Yet, within that universe, there are constellations, stars, and moons. We have some certainty about these fixed points within that space. In medicine, the fixed points are studies and trials that provide the 'evidence base'.

When faced with an individual patient, it is our role to best fit our knowledge of that universe of information to the individual. We may align the stars of knowledge into Orion for a particular patient. For another, we may rearrange those stars of knowledge to a different constellation, perhaps Capricorn, Aquarius or the Big Dipper.

Our reality is that the human body (the universe) is currently beyond our comprehension, and our gaps in knowledge (the nothingness between the planets and the stars) are profound.

a change in approach

What if we could identify patients who were going to have a heart attack early and start preventative therapy before they have their coronary event?

This approach would require us to be far more precise in our evaluation of the individual and far less reliant on that individual's risk within a population.

The medical classification refers to 'low risk' as up to a 10 per cent chance within 10 years and does not consider treatment.

This could be expressed as a one per cent chance per annum of having a major event.

Would you find the same risk acceptable if you applied it to air travel?

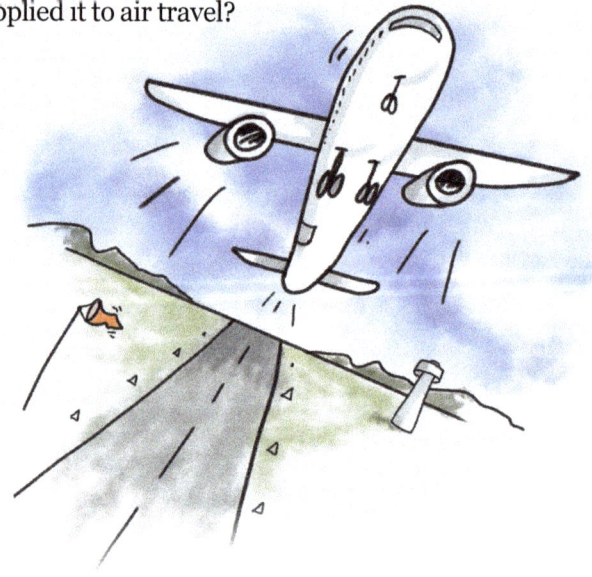

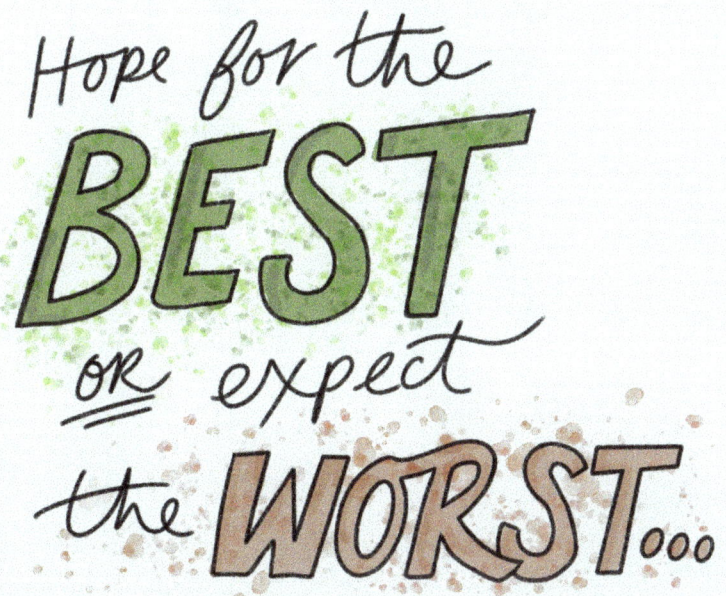

We don't routinely treat individuals in a low-risk population, although up to 10 per cent of this cohort may have an event. This is the hope for the best as some of those individuals will have a MACE (major adverse coronary event). Let's hope it is not someone we have reassured!

Conversely, we treat all individuals in a high-risk population, although up to 80 per cent of them will have no problem at all in the next 10 years. This is expecting the worst.

IMPORTANT POINTS

BEING AHEAD OF THE GAME

- Risk management, historically, focuses on secondary prevention, after the first heart event has occurred. We believe that primary prevention (treatment for risk before an event) could be used more effectively, and save lives.
- Risk prevention is individual and takes many factors into consideration.
- Imaging can improve risk prediction.
- The earlier risk factors are treated, the better the patient's outcome.

---

16 Kannel WB, McGee D, Gordon T. A general cardiovascular risk profile: The Framingham study. *The American Journal of Cardiology* 1978; 38:46-51.

17 Greenland P, LaBree L, Azen SP, Doherty TM, Detrano RC. Coronary artery calcium score combined with Framingham score for risk prediction in asymptomatic individuals. *Jama* 2004; 291:210-5.

As we move forward in our discussion about preventing heart attacks, there are two key perspectives that will underpin our discussion:

- *your lifestyle choices, and*
- *knowing your risk through a more precise mechanism than assessment using a population-based tool.*

Let's look at the 10 commandments for risk reduction.

10 COMMANDMENTS OF HEART HEALTH

1. Don't smoke.
2. Exercise regularly for your physical and mental health
3. Eat well, maintain a healthy weight.
4. Limit alcohol consumption.
5. Keep blood pressure under control.
6. Be on top of diabetes.
7. Know your cardiovascular risk. Precisely.
8. Know your cholesterol level and act on it.
9. Understand aspirin and other heart medications.
10. Have a team to support you with your health objectives.

Start as early in life as you can to implement these steps. Small investments early pay huge, cumulative dividends.

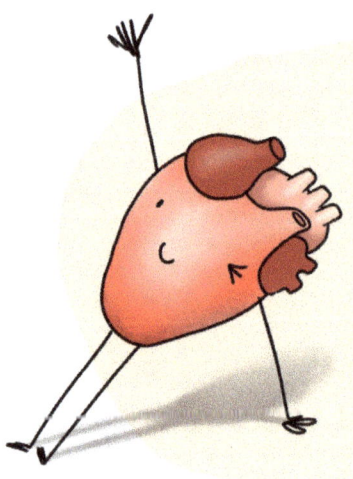

Change is possible, especially:

- ☒ with the help of education
- ☒ through seeking medical advice
- ☒ asking for the support and encouragement of others.

chapter 4
THE 10 COMMANDMENTS

Earlier, we talked about the categorisation of heart attack risk as 'low', 'intermediate', or 'high'. The likelihood of an event occurring in the next five or 10 years is associated with various health-related behaviours, illnesses, and societal factors. These include behavioural and biomedical factors, as well as socio-economic, environmental, and other influences. Most risk factors can be changed through lifestyle modifications, but some, such as family history, age, gender, and ethnicity, cannot be altered. Additionally, as mentioned in the previous chapter, there are certain features that currently remain unexplained.

Heart attack and angina are the two major clinical forms of **coronary heart disease** (CHD), one of several cardiac diseases under the umbrella term **cardiovascular disease** (CVD), which refers to all diseases of the heart and blood vessels as a consequence of diseased arteries.

Atherosclerosis (plaque build-up in the coronary arteries) – often called 'hardening of the arteries' – is the underlying process behind CVD. As we have already seen, arteries can clog with plaque. When it affects the blood supply to

- the **heart**, angina (partial blockage) or a heart attack (complete blockage) results;
- the **brain**, a stroke is the outcome;
- the **legs/feet**, peripheral vascular disease can be the consequence.

Risk factors are often considered in isolation. However, while risk factors are independent predictors of disease – that is, the presence of each one on its own increases the risk of illness – they also have an interactive effect. The presence of additional risk factors increases the risk of illness. While it is never too late to start, the earlier you begin eliminating modifiable risk factors from your life, the better your long-term health outcome.

You can't live for five, six or seven decades and expect your 'investment' – or lack of 'investment' – in your health won't impact your more senior years.

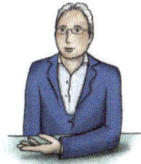

In our attempt to prevent heart attack, let us look at the 10 commandments for a healthier heart. The 'headline' of each 'commandment' follows, giving an overview. Subsequent chapters will flesh out the details.

commandment 1 – don't smoke

Don't smoke – please!

Please do whatever you can to quit any form of smoking, including passive smoking, nicotine replacement, vaping and using snuff. Find whatever support is necessary. **Smoking is a curse**. Most people, on average, need about six attempts to quit smoking and maintain it.

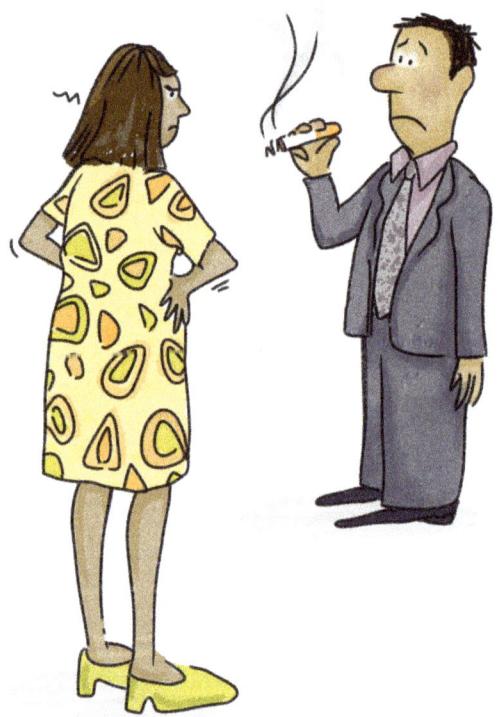

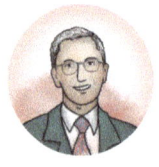

If you've tried once, twice, or thrice to give up smoking, you've got three more times to try before you're even at the average! So please, please, please **don't quit quitting**[18].

commandment 2 – exercise regularly for your physical and mental health

All studies examining exercise and cardiovascular outcomes show that **exercise is beneficial**. Similarly, studies also link mental health and cardio health. The question then becomes, *How much?* The recommendation is at least five sessions of 30 minutes per week of at least moderate exercise, so maybe walking briskly[19]. If you have a step counter, walking 10,000 steps is a great daily goal, although more than 8000 will offer a similar benefit.

For most people to maintain exercise and develop it into a **habit**, the activity also should be **enjoyable**. So, find something that gives you pleasure as well.

Regular exercise aids good **mental health** as it can help reduce stress, anxiety, and depression by releasing endorphins and improving cognitive function. It also provides an opportunity for social interaction and a sense of accomplishment, which can improve self-esteem and overall well-being.

commandment 3 – eat well, maintain a healthy weight

We know we should eat a healthy diet (no question), but there is a deal of confusion about a sound approach.

It is straightforward.

Avoid food in packets with barcodes and food that does not spoil when exposed to air.

Mixed grains, fruit and nuts are good.

Legumes, such as pulses and beans, are fantastic, as is garlic.

Keep saturated fats and processed foods to a minimum. For example, meats such as salamis and bacon are high in saturated fats and other preservatives, which are not good.

Dr Bishop has a weight loss program:
https://drwarrickbishop.com/s/tfbsg

Refined sugar offers no benefit, so sweets, pastries, baked delicacies, and sugary drinks should not be in your diet.

Maintaining a healthy weight is essential. If you drift, the sooner you can get onto it, the better. Controlling weight might be where some team members come into play – a dietitian, a local doctor and/or friends or family. Decide to alter calories, reduce carbohydrates, and walk more.

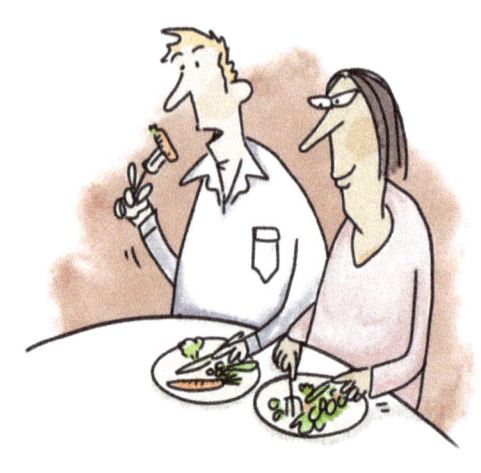

commandment 4 – limit your alcohol consumption

The bloodstream absorbs alcohol while the alcohol is being consumed, and is distributed throughout the body, temporarily elevating the heart rate and blood pressure. Consistently drinking in excess is strongly associated with persistent elevated blood pressure, which can exert pressure on the heart. This increased pressure can cause cardiovascular disease, escalating the likelihood of the drinker experiencing a heart attack or stroke.

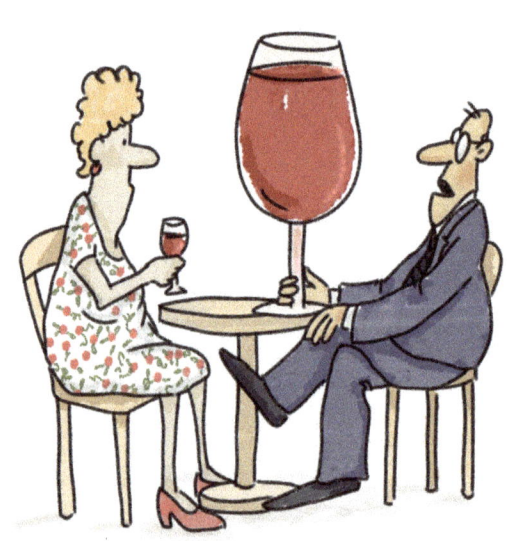

Moreover, prolonged alcohol abuse can result in narrowed arteries due to atherosclerosis, a weakened heart muscle, and atrial fibrillation, which all contribute to a higher risk of heart attack and stroke.[20]

Now I've turned 50, I've been limiting myself to one glass a day. It seems to be going well.

commandment 5 – keep your blood pressure under control

High blood pressure links closely to heart attack, stroke, cardiac failure (CF), atrial fibrillation (AF), and renal impairment. Increasing amounts of data suggest an association with Alzheimer's disease.

Initial blood pressure treatment should focus on non-pharmacological (non-drug) means such as weight loss and exercise. Both are powerful in reducing blood pressure. Excessive alcohol consumption can also have a significant negative impact on a person's blood pressure levels.

commandment 6 – be on top of diabetes

Type 2 diabetes and pre-diabetes[21] are major risk factors in relation to cardiac events.

Although significant, both conditions can be managed – reduced or reversed – by lifestyle modification, mainly through diet, aided by establishing clear, well-guided habits, including exercise.

Reducing carbohydrates is a great start, and regular exercise will burn up the sugars in the bloodstream. Both will help with weight loss. And weight loss is critical to managing diabetes and pre-diabetes – and the sooner, the better. Medications, both established and new, are also available if needed.

commandment 7 – know your cardiovascular risk – precisely

You should know and understand your risk of a heart attack, particularly if you are an adult between your mid-40s and 75 years of age, have a family history of 'early' heart disease or live with several cardiovascular risk factors. Our strong recommendation is that you have your risk assessed.

Risk calculators have been developed, and you should discuss them with your doctor. Specific conversations about what is going on for you, the individual, guide precise prevention or treatment plans:

- Would a blood pressure medication alter your risk?
- Would a cholesterol medication lessen your risk?
- Do you need to take aspirin regularly to lower your risk?

Such discussions **must** be with your **doctor**, not Dr Google or some well-meaning family member or friend. **Follow-up** is needed regularly.

For many people, risk assessment benefits from imaging the heart. This process starts with a coronary artery calcium (CAC) score, which measures the amount of calcified plaque in the arteries. Further explanation can be found in chapter 11.

All risk assessment builds to a more accurate knowledge of a person's situation rather than simply being a probability. This knowledge leads to more precise preventative treatments being available – for you.

commandment 8 – know your cholesterol level and act on it

Current Western world guidelines flag elevated cholesterol – specifically high LDL or 'bad' cholesterol – as needing treatment using cholesterol-lowering medications to reduce the risk of heart attack or stroke. The most used cholesterol-lowering agents are statins.

Individuals should know their LDL levels, targets and how to achieve them.

LDL targets depend on **personal** risk. For patients who have not had an event (that is, as a primary prevention measure), an LDL level of 2.5 millimoles[22] per litre may be sufficient. However, for patients who are at high risk – as identified by imaging or who have had a heart attack or stroke – (as a secondary prevention measure) much lower levels (<1.4 mmo/l) are recommended and can be achieved.

The first steps, diet and lifestyle, are foundational and have a modest effect. Medications, including statins, ezetimibe, and PCSK9 inhibitors *(to be discussed later)*, often in combination, can reduce LDL by up to 80 per cent. Neutraceuticals can also be beneficial. Consultation with your GP and cardiologist will lead to the best strategy to lower your LDL cholesterol level to meet your target.

commandment 9 – understand aspirin and other heart medications

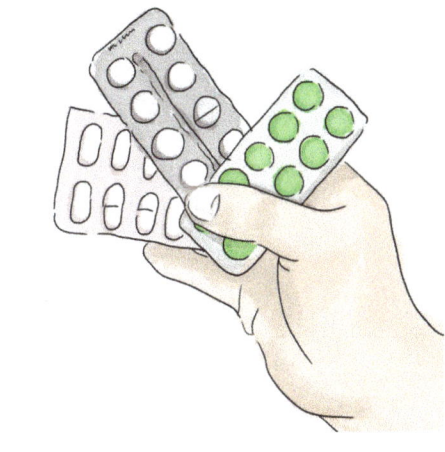

Using aspirin regularly is **not** for everyone, and aspirin should **not** be self-prescribed. The literature says that decisions must be precise regarding who should use it. You must discuss its risk – increased bleeding – with your doctor or specialist. Does its benefit to you outweigh this risk? Generally, it is routinely prescribed in secondary prevention as these patients are at high risk of another cardiac event. The use of imaging can help inform this decision-making in the primary prevention setting.

Importantly, continue to take your medications. They only work when you do!

commandment 10 – have a team to support you

Optimum health care, and especially heart health, is not solo travel. You will engage with your local family doctor and, perhaps, a specialist.

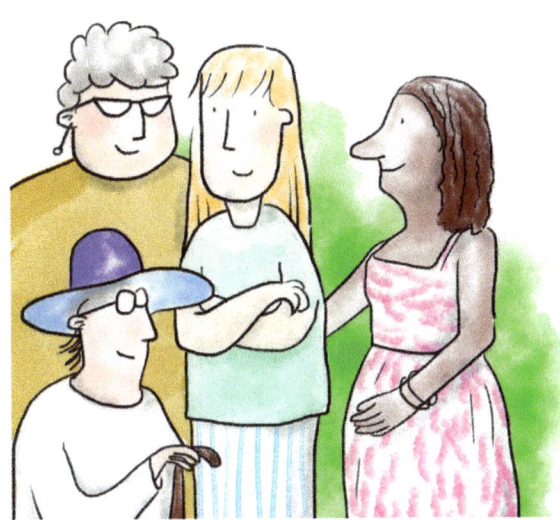

Others on the team could include your significant other, a dietitian, and an exercise physiologist. As it is well recognised that socio-economic issues can significantly impact a person's cardiovascular health, consider including a social worker on your team. And don't forget your supportive partner, family, and friends.

start early

The underpinning message from these 10 commandments is to **start reducing your risk early**. Small investments as early as possible pay the most considerable dividends in the longer term as they provide cumulative benefits. If you live without attention to these cardiovascular health commandments, you cannot rely on miraculous change 'at the last minute'.

These commandments are fleshed out in the following pages, giving you **encouragement**, **information** and **resources** that will help you start with small but sure steps as the best way to look after yourself and your heart. Such self-care will help

- avoid coronary artery disease – particularly a heart attack
- improve general health
- reduce the risk of cancer and dementia, and support an improved quality of life.

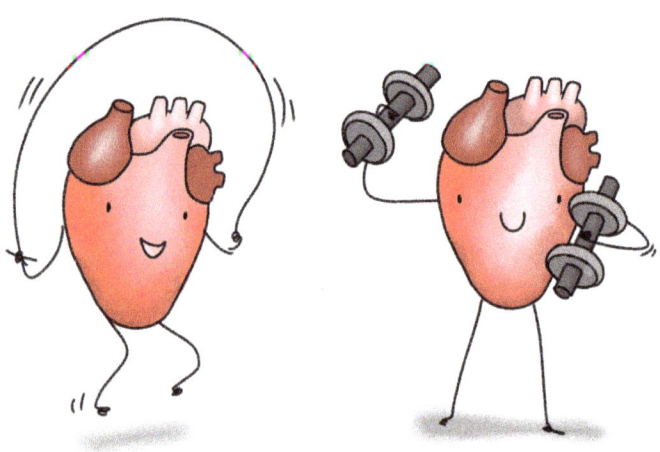

IMPORTANT POINTS

THE 10 COMMANDMENTS

- There are 10 commandments to help reduce risk of a heart attack:
  1. Don't smoke.
  2. Exercise regularly for your physical and mental health.
  3. Eat well, maintain a healthy weight.
  4. Limit your alcohol consumption.
  5. Keep your blood pressure under control.
  6. Be on top of diabetes.
  7. Know your cardiovascular risk – precisely.
  8. Know your cholesterol level and act on it.
  9. Understand aspirin and other heart medications.
  10. Have a team to support you with your health objectives.
- Start as early in life as you can to implement these steps. Small investments early pay huge, cumulative dividends.
- Even if you have missed the 'early boat', it is never too late to start.

---

18 A phrase taken from a long-running QUIT advertising campaign in Australia.
19 https://www.heartfoundation.org.au/Heart-health-education/physical-activity-and-exercise
20 based on material from the Heart Research Institute (https://www.hri.org.au/)
21 Before diabetes; when a person's sugar levels are drifting up and weight is settling around the tummy.
22 A mole is an amount of substance that contains a large number – 6 followed by 23 zeros – of molecules or atoms. One millimole is 1/1000th of a mole.

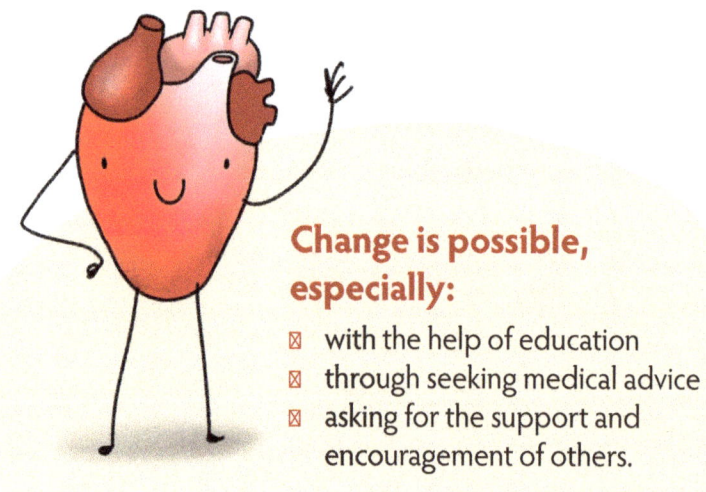

Change is possible, especially:

- with the help of education
- through seeking medical advice
- asking for the support and encouragement of others.

Please! Please! Please! Do not smoke!

chapter 5
QUIT! QUIT! QUIT!

 SMOKING – Smoking is the single leading cause of preventable mortality and morbidity, affecting nearly all body systems and increasing the risk of a multitude of diseases, including cardiovascular disease, cancer, respiratory disease, chronic kidney disease, dementia, and diabetes.

Smoking cessation reduces the risk of non-communicable diseases and prevents a wide variety of other chronic and acute health conditions...

VAPING – Cessation of nicotine and/or non-nicotine vaping should be strongly encouraged as there are inherent health risks in repeatedly inhaling the aerosol (with and without nicotine). Evidence is emerging that vaping nicotine increases blood pressure, heart rate and arterial stiffness. This could potentially increase the risk of developing cardiovascular disease and compromised lung function. Vaping products can also potentially cause accidental and intentional poisonings (including deaths), seizures, burns and injuries.

SMOKING AND VAPING FROM *QUIT AND HEART FOUNDATION POSITION STATEMENT: SMOKING AND VAPING CESSATION, SEPTEMBER 2021*[23]

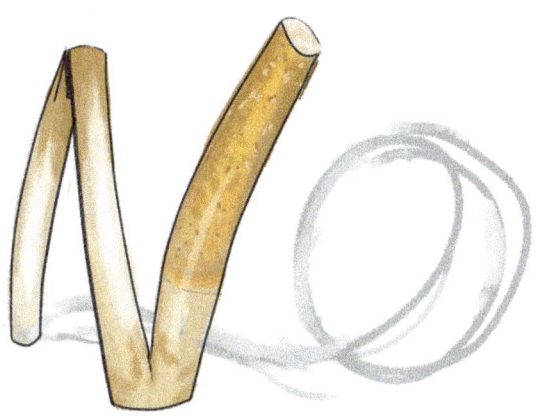

> **E-CIGARETTES** – Electronic nicotine delivery systems such as e-cigarettes have been developed and advertised as safer alternatives to traditional tobacco cigarettes. Aggressive marketing strategies and misleading claims by manufacturers have largely contributed to the belief that e-cigarettes are harmless. In reality, e-cigarettes are far from innocuous. E-cigarette solutions and aerosols generally contain harmful substances that are commonly found in tobacco cigarette emissions. A growing body of literature suggests that e-cigarettes are associated with an increased risk of cardiovascular morbidity and mortality. In addition, the effectiveness of e-cigarettes as smoking cessation tools has yet to be determined. Concerningly, most smokers do not give up on tobacco cigarettes and eventually become dual users.
>
> *E-CIGARETTES: A NEW THREAT TO CARDIOVASCULAR HEALTH, A WORLD HEART FEDERATION POLICY BRIEF, OCTOBER 2021*[24]

Australia records more than 20,000 deaths caused by smoking every year[25]. **Tobacco** smoke is one of the main risk factors for heart disease and is responsible for 12 per cent of Australia's cardiovascular disease burden (death and illness)[26]. The World Heart Federation puts this figure at 17 per cent globally[27].

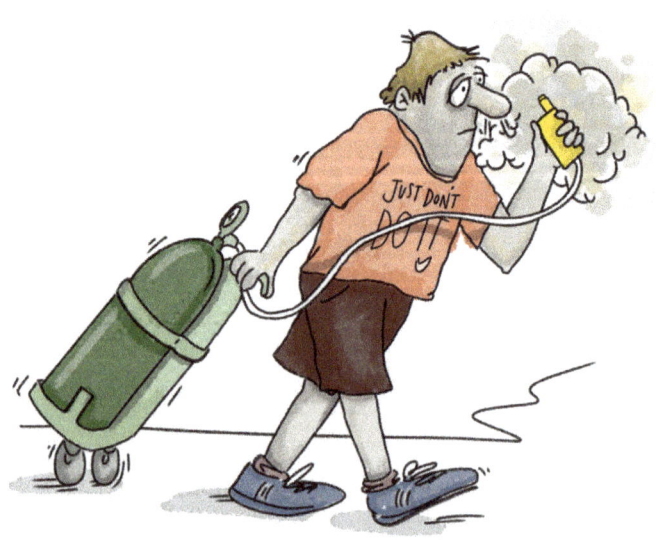

no good news

As you already know, no good news exists about tobacco and smoking.

Smoking – which includes passive smoking, chewing tobacco, vaping (using an e-cigarette) and snuff –

- damages the lining of the blood vessels (the endothelium),
- can cause a stiffening of the blood vessels,
- increases fatty deposits in the arteries,
- contributes to atherosclerosis (narrowing and clogging of the arteries),
- increases the risk of blood clotting,
- affects cholesterol and triglyceride levels,
- promotes coronary artery spasm (a temporary tightening of the muscles in the wall of an artery that can reduce or block blood flow to part of the heart),
- accelerates heart rate, and
- increases blood pressure.

None of these problems is good for the heart.

Smokers suffer more heart attacks, strokes, and angina than non-smokers, **and** at a much younger age. A smoker is four times more likely to die of heart disease (i.e., heart attack or stroke) and three times more likely to die from sudden cardiac death than a non-smoker [28].

Smoking kills 17 Australians every day through cardiovascular diseases such as heart attack and stroke.[29] Women who smoke are at a higher risk of heart attack than men who smoke.

Smoking is arguably the leading preventable cause of mortality and morbidity in the western world. Therefore, mitigating future risk by smoking cessation is a powerful objective. Not only does it affect your heart, but it also impacts your lungs in terms of breathing effectiveness and opens the risk of cancer in the lungs, mouth and oesophagus, as well as peripheral vascular disease, and skin problems.

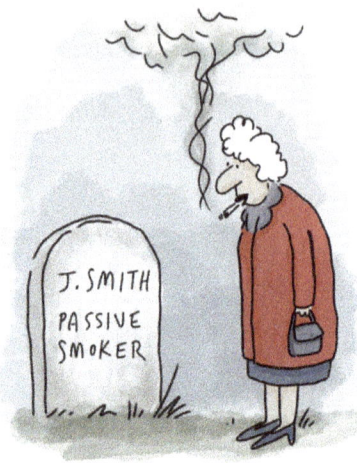

beyond cigarettes

Unfortunately, the news is bad not only for the smoker but also for **passive smokers** – loved ones, friends, and colleagues.

Passive, or second-hand, cigarette smoke impact is significant, including on unborn children. Considerable exposure to second-hand smoke can have the same consequences as being the smoker.

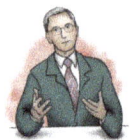

*So, **smokers**, please be considerate of others. And if you are in a **passive** smoking situation, please have the necessary conversations to look after your health.*

e-cigarettes

And if you are hoping for some help through e-cigarettes, please **avoid** them. Not much long-term data are available, but preliminary indicators are that the body treats e-cigarette chemicals **the same way as a standard cigarette.**

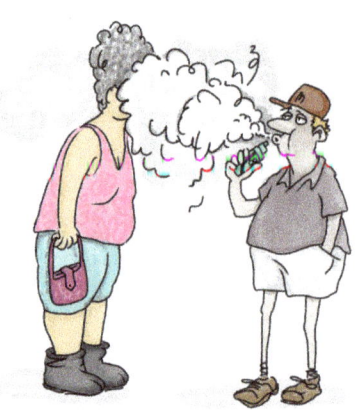

If you are a smoker, please do whatever you can to put it behind you. After stopping for two years, the risk of heart attack returns to that of a matched non-smoking cohort – a good return on your 'investment'.

doesn't take much

Smokers only need a couple of cigarettes a day to keep their risks elevated – risks of heart attack, stroke, cancer. Cutting down is a great **start** – and it may slow progress to lung disease – but it **doesn't** completely reduce your risk. For that, you need to **stop smoking**.

planning, persistence, patience

Quitting smoking is not an easy thing to do. Few people can go 'cold turkey', unless, of course, they are in a coronary care unit recovering from a heart attack. For most people, it requires **planning**, **persistence**, and **patience** – and a **genuine desire** to change. Such desire goes beyond head knowledge; beyond even the recognition that smoking has contributed to your current state of health and is a real danger in the future.

Advice from your cardiologist and general practitioner can be very effective in modifying smoking behaviours. General practitioners are important here as they see patients more frequently than the cardiologist and can coach the patient.

Nicotine replacement has helped many people quit. Programs such as QuitLine[30] can also provide terrific advice and encouragement.

Although smoking causes severe damage, over time, stopping smoking effectively reduces cardiovascular risk to close to that of a person who has not smoked.[31] Quitting smoking also protects the health of your family, friends, and colleagues and has the added advantage of saving money, as in most parts of the world, it is a costly habit.

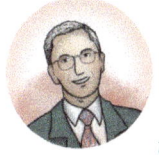

If you really must have the occasional puff, limit yourself to cigars at weddings and births and don't inhale. Pass it around and enjoy the day. Do your best to put the cigarettes and smoking behind you so you can enjoy improved health.

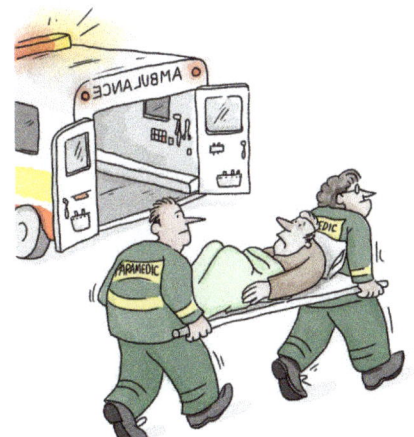

IMPORTANT POINTS

QUIT!

- Quitting smoking has an almost immediate positive effect on your risk of heart attack and stroke; this positive effect increases significantly over time.
- Be especially aware of the dangers of
  - e-cigarettes
  - passive smoking on others.
- Programs are very helpful when trying to quit smoking.
- General practitioners, in particular, and cardiologists have a role to play in educating and supporting patients to quit smoking.
- Quitting is a great money saver.

---

23   Position statement https://www.heartfoundation.org.au/getmedia/cd93970f-7b17-4e35-96f8-665557089f81/Quit-HeartFoundation-Position-Statement-October-2021.pdf

24   Bianco E, Skipalskyi A, Goma F, Odeh H, Hasegawa K, Al-Zawawi M, Stoklosa M, Dalmau R, Dorotheo EU, et al. E-Cigarettes: A New Threat to Cardiovascular Health – A World Heart Federation Policy Brief. Global Heart. Oct 2021; 16(1): 72. DOI: https://doi.org/10.5334/gh.1076

25   Heart Foundation (Australia) https://www.heartfoundation.org.au/Programs/Advocacy-Smoking-and-tobacco-regulation

26   ibid.

27   World Heart Federation https://world-heart-federation.org/wp-content/uploads/E-cigarettes-Policy-Brief.pdf p4

28   Heart Foundation (Australia) website https://www.heartfoundation.org.au/Heart-health-education/Smoking-and-your-heart

29   Heart Research Institute: https://www.hri.org.au (health/learn/risk factors/smoking)

30   Australia. Each country will have a variety of programs available.

31   World Heart Federation website: https://world-heart-federation.org/ What can you do to lower your risk of cardiovascular disease?

We know that exercise is good for us and, yet, so often we resist it.

chapter 6
BODY AND MIND

PHYSICAL VITALITY

 Exercise is a celebration of what your body can do, not a punishment for what you ate. ... exercise with variety and regularity. I promise you'll be the happiest, healthiest version of yourself.

ALICIA PHILIPATOS[32]

You know – everyone knows – that exercise is good for you. And we know that exercise comes in two main types:

aerobic exercise (for example, walking along a beach, swinging your arms and moving your legs freely, where your heart rate goes up)

and

resistance exercise (holding, bracing, or lifting a weight).

Despite knowing that exercise is good, about 50 per cent of adults in the western world do not exercise as much as they should, falling well short of current national and international recommendations.

Encouragingly, 'exercise' includes everyday activities such as walking to the shops or taking the stairs, as well as more organised movement, including sports, walking groups, yoga or attending a gym. Maybe even more importantly, it includes activities that you already enjoy. And the other good news is that **anyone** can increase physical activity at **any age** and from **any fitness level**.

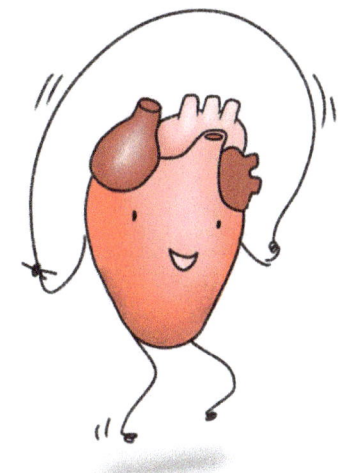

WONDER DRUG – The Heart Foundation calls walking the 'wonder drug'.[33] Walking for an average of 30 minutes or more a day can lower the risk of heart disease, stroke by 35 per cent and type 2 diabetes by 40 per cent.

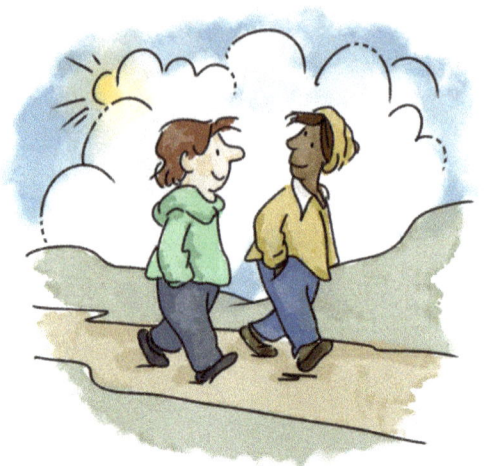

exercise recommendations

The medical fraternity recommends that individuals undertake about 150 minutes per week of **moderate intensity** exercise (the heart rate increases but not to the point of breathlessness). That could be a walk. You could try something like this: a 15-minute walk to and from your car or public transport on your work commute would give you 30 minutes a day, five days a week, and there are your 150 minutes.

We recognise, too, that **higher intensity** exercise has a greater benefit. Guidelines suggest about 75 minutes of high-intensity exercise. That might be running three 25-minute runs in a week.

You should incorporate **balance** and **flexibility** exercises on most days and include specific **strength** exercises on two-to-three days of the week.

And don't sit for too long, regardless of whether you are at work or home. **Sedentary behaviour is a big problem**. The evidence says that many CVD patients engage in high levels of sedentary behaviour.[34] Additionally, the evidence shows that CVD patients with a more sedentary lifestyle are at increased risk of premature mortality (death).[35]

Australia's Heart Foundation splits its recommendations into age groups: babies to 5 years of age, 5 to 17 years, 18 to 64 years and 65 years and older.[36]

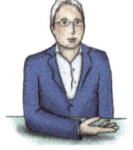

Please don't miss the chance to be active. Do what you do with some frequency and regularity. Stay happy, stay healthy, and stay exercising!

benefits

Regular exercise is as effective as antidepressant medication for mood.[37] And so begins a list of significant benefits that not only assist heart health by reducing the risk of heart disease and heart attacks but also incorporates prevention and management of a range of conditions and diseases that include some cancers, type 2 diabetes and depression.

Specifically, it helps with weight control. If someone starts to exercise for weight loss, the weight shed often is from around the tummy ('hazardous waste') and the waist circumference decreases. This loss links closely with a reduced risk of heart attack in the future.

Exercise will help reduce blood pressure and improve insulin resistance, meaning that the body deals with sugars and carbohydrates more effectively. It also changes the cholesterol balances within the bloodstream, raising 'good' cholesterol and lowering 'bad' cholesterol.

just do it

Whatever you do, put **exercise into your daily routine**. Think about where you can increase incidental exercise around your daily activities:

- park the car away from your destination
- take the stairs instead of the lift
- 'lose' the remote control
- stretch rather than stand on a step
- dance during commercial breaks
- pace while you are on the phone
- set a phone reminder to stand up and move every hour.

Find something you enjoy. My experience (WB) is you can't tell people to **go** cycling, **go** walking, **go** running, **go** swimming because if it is not enjoyable to the person, it won't be sustainable. As this is long-haul rather than quick-fix, please find something you enjoy:

- wade through a pool with your friends – **great**;
- take up jazzercise – **amazing**;

- walk along a beach (at sunrise/sunset) – **romantic**;
- run if your knees and hips are good – **excellent**;
- cycle, but please wear bright coloured clothes and preferably use cycling tracks – **marvellous**.

Walking is known to have many health benefits. Some studies suggest that a leisurely walk after eating is beneficial. Although sufferers of high blood pressure and diabetes receive special mention here, the results suggest that enjoying a short, light-intensity walk after a meal improves health, even for a healthy person.[38]

Whatever you do, increase your activity because not only does exercise help with your weight, blood pressure and cholesterol levels, good data show that exercise is good for mood – as good as a mild anti-depressive agent. The benefit is cumulative.

 Exercise is medicine.

ROBERT ZECCHIN[39]

HEAT SHOCK PROTEINS

Several years ago, I (WB) attended a meeting where a presenter spoke about the development of heat shock proteins. These proteins respond to the physical effort, the stress and the strain put on the muscles by exercise. A knock-on effect is that these proteins have metabolic effects such as increasing metabolism and reducing insulin resistance.

The fascinating thing, however, is that temperature activates these heat shock proteins. You can receive similar exercise benefits from having a 30-minute hot bath or even a 30-minute sauna. It sounds like a luxurious way to get in your 150 minutes per week!

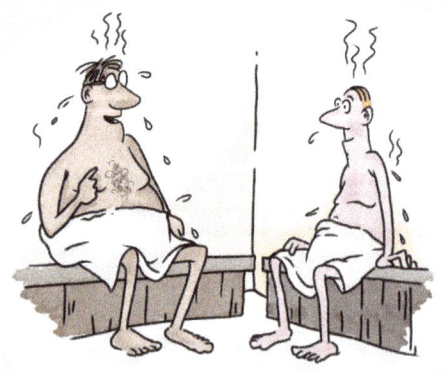

MENTAL WELL-BEING

> *(Cardiovascular disease – CVD) should not be addressed as an isolated entity, but rather as one part of an integrated system, in which mind, heart, and body are interconnected. Both positive psychological status and negative psychological status appear to affect cardiovascular health and prognosis directly. Wellness and well-being involve not only physical factors but also psychological ones. Clinicians should strive to treat not just the disease state but the patient ... as a whole.*
>
> **FROM A STATEMENT BY THE AMERICAN HEART ASSOCIATION ISSUED IN JANUARY 2021**[40]

In relation to the heart, mental health embraces two key aspects: maintaining a strong mental state in daily life and addressing the psychological impact after experiencing a heart event or receiving a diagnosis.

interconnection

The mind and the heart are linked[41]. A person's emotional well-being can profoundly influence that person's cardiovascular health. Here are several compelling reasons why maintaining robust mental health is crucial to your heart's health:

- **stress reduction**: High levels of stress can lead to increased cortisol levels and inflammation in the body, which are associated with a higher risk of heart disease. Good mental health practices, such as mindfulness and relaxation techniques, can help manage stress and promote a healthier heart.
- **healthy lifestyle choices**: Individuals with strong mental health are more likely to make positive lifestyle choices. They are motivated to exercise regularly, maintain a balanced diet, avoid smoking, and limit alcohol consumption – all of which are essential for heart health.
- **adherence to medical treatments**: People with better mental well-being are more likely to adhere to prescribed medical treatments and follow advice, leading to better ongoing health outcomes.

- **social support**: Good mental health fosters positive social interactions and strong support networks, which can buffer against the negative effects of stress.
- **emotional regulation**: Being able to cope with emotions effectively can prevent emotional stressors from having a detrimental impact on heart health. Poor mental health, on the other hand, can lead to behaviours that increase the risk of heart disease, such as emotional eating or substance abuse.
- **improved sleep**: Better sleep patterns and sufficient rest are crucial for cardiovascular health and the body's ability to repair itself.

detrimental processes		beneficial processes	
• stress, anxiety, depression • pessimism • smoking initiation • physical inactivity	• poor- and over-eating • weight gain • medication non-compliance	• equanimity, happiness • optimism • smoking cessation • increased physical activity • heart, healthy eating	• weight loss • blood pressure reduction • disease mgt / medication compliance
biological processes		**biological processes**	
• increased inflammation	• higher LDL • higher BP	• decreased inflammation • lower LDL	• lower BP
CV health		**CV health**	
• increased CV risk factors	• increased incident CVD	• reduced CV risk factors • decreased incident CVD	• secondary prevention

psychological health (healthy mind)

Here are five practices that promote and support well-being and quality of life as they can enhance self-awareness and effectively assist in handling negative thoughts and emotions.

- **regular exercise**: We have already seen that engaging in physical activity not only benefits the body but also positively impacts mental health. Regular exercise triggers the release of endorphins, which naturally uplift the mood and help alleviate stress and anxiety. Whether it's walking, jogging, yoga, or any other form of exercise, staying active can enhance mood and promote mental well-being.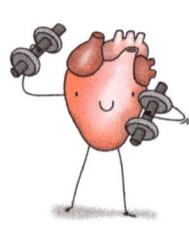
- **mindfulness and meditation**: Incorporating mindfulness and meditation into daily routines can aid in stress reduction and induce relaxation.

- Mindfulness entails being fully immersed in the present moment without passing judgment, while
- meditation fosters mental clarity, relaxation, and inner peace.

- **social connections**: Maintain strong social connections and nurturing relationships are important. Engaging with friends, family, or participating in community activities can provide a sense of belonging and support during challenging times. Social interactions also contribute to positive emotions and a sense of fulfillment.
- **balanced diet**: Eating a nutritious and balanced diet is not only important for physical health but also impacts mental well-being.
  - Consuming a variety of fruits, vegetables, whole grains, and healthy fats can provide essential nutrients that support brain health.
  - Avoiding excessive caffeine, alcohol, and processed foods can also contribute to better mental health.
- **self-care and stress management**: Taking time for self-care is essential. Engaging in activities that bring joy and relaxation, such as reading, hobbies, or spending time in nature, can rejuvenate the mind. Additionally, learning effective stress management techniques, such as deep breathing exercises or journaling, can help cope with life's challenges and reduce the impact of stress on mental health.

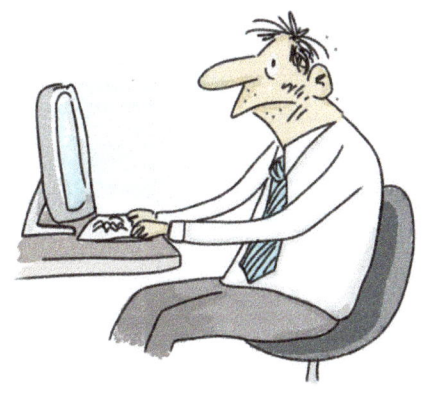

Remember, your journey to good mental health is unique. It is essential to find practices that resonate with you, personally.

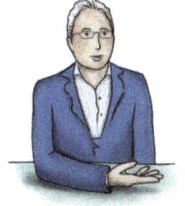

If necessary, seek professional help. Giving importance to mental health contributes not only to personal well-being but also to overall happiness and fulfillment in life.

psychological impact

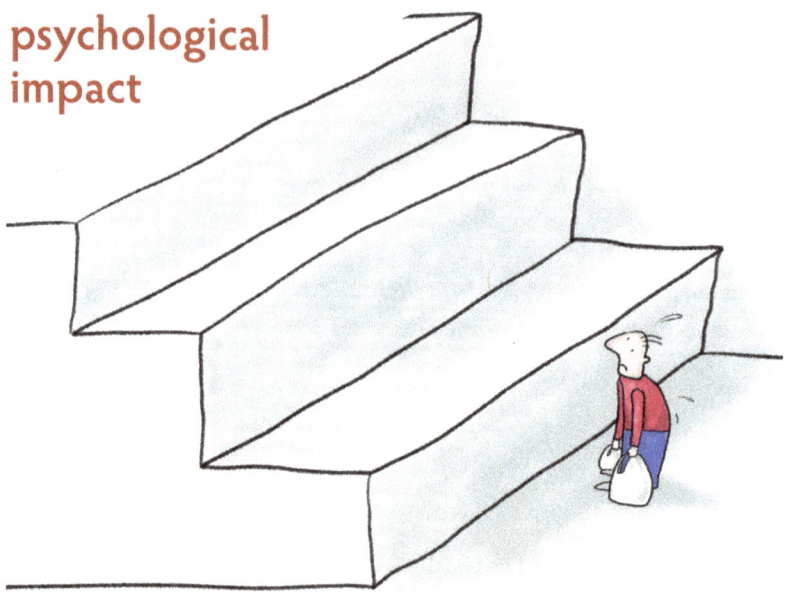

Experiencing a heart attack, other heart event or receiving a heart-related diagnosis can have significant psychological implications. Here are five points that highlight the potential inner impact:

- **emotional distress**: A heart event or diagnosis can trigger a range of emotions such as fear, anxiety, sadness, or even shock. Dealing with the uncertainty of the condition and potential lifestyle changes can lead to emotional distress and feelings of vulnerability.

- **depression and anxiety**: The psychological impact of an event or diagnosis may increase the risk of developing depression and anxiety. Patients may worry about their prognosis, future health, and the potential limitations on their daily activities.

- **adjustment difficulties**: Coping with the aftermath of a heart event or diagnosis can be challenging as it often requires adapting to a 'new reality' of lifestyle modifications, medication regimens, medical procedures, new medical practitioners. Overwhelming!

- **self-esteem and body image**: Changes in physical health, such as weight loss, scars from surgeries, or restrictions in physical abilities, can influence a person's self-esteem and body image. This may lead to feelings of insecurity or a sense of loss of control over one's body.

- **impact on relationships**: Relationships with family, friends, or partners also can be affected. Patients may experience changes in their roles within the family or social circle, and loved ones may also struggle to cope with the emotional aspects of the situation.

It is essential for individuals experiencing the psychological impact of a heart event or diagnosis to seek support from healthcare professionals, counsellors, or support groups. Addressing the emotional aspects of the condition can significantly improve overall well-being and aid in the rate and degree of recovery[42].

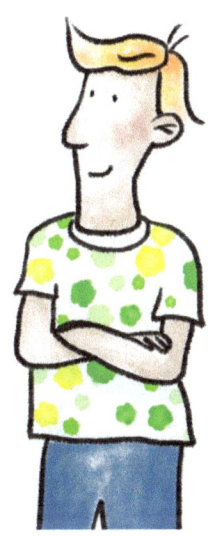

Dr Bishop, as part of his Healthy Heart Network, has a fascinating and far-ranging podcast interview[43] with a liaison psychiatrist, Dr Ralf Ilchef, who is Director of Liaison Psychiatry at Royal North Shore Hospital, Sydney, Australia. The interview is also reproduced in Dr Bishop's book, *Cardiac Rehabilitation Explained* (2023).

Dr Ralf Ilchef: There's nothing like a major cardiac event to make people have a reset in their life and to do what they can do to resume control of their life, improve their physical health, improve their relationships. Think about the impact of depression and anxiety. We've talked so far about heart disease predisposing people to depression, but it's important to know that depression predisposes you to heart disease. So, people living with depression are putting themselves at risk. Mental health is always something that you want to optimise ... So, it's a great opportunity to really give yourself a 20,000-kilometre service and have your mental and emotional health seen to along with your physical health.

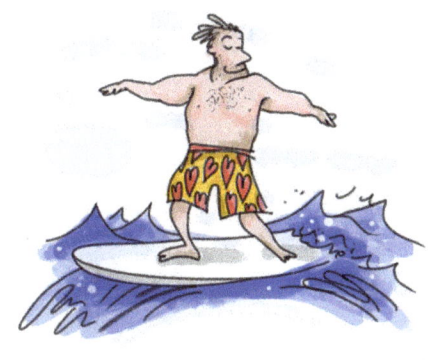

find an exercise that is not a chore

And remember, there's never been a better time to have a cardiac event. Medicine has come such a long way. There are so many wonderful treatments available, and more coming down the tube, so that people should feel confident that they have never been better placed to have a good outcome from a cardiac event – to be confident that they have a lot of life ahead of them, and that they should live it as well as they can ...

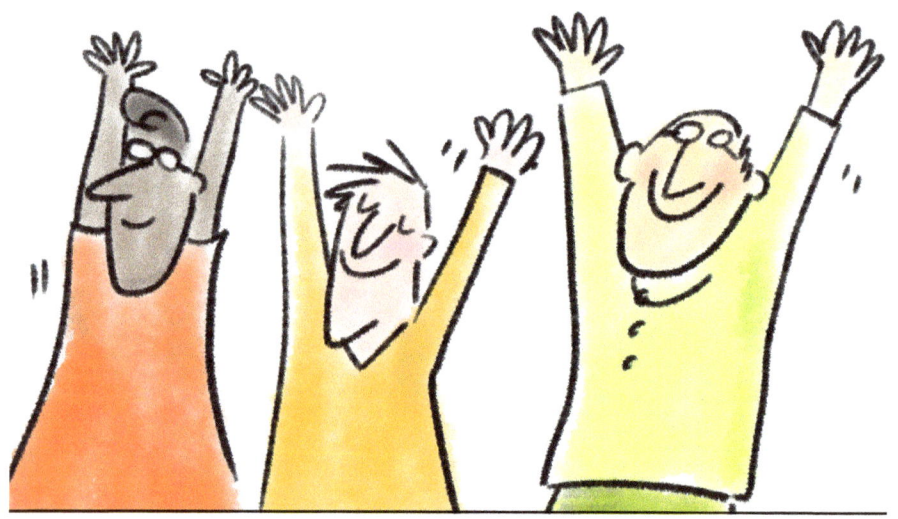

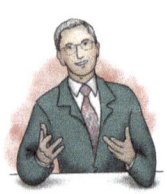

So, strong mental health is not only essential for emotional well-being but also a vital factor in maintaining heart health. Practicing self-care, stress management, and seeking support when needed can lead to a healthier mind-heart connection and a reduced risk of cardiovascular disease, and, in particular, heart attack.

IMPORTANT POINTS

BODY AND MIND

Physical Vitality

- Regular exercise
  - is as effective as anti-depressant medication for depression
  - benefits and helps manage heart health
  - benefits and helps manage other health conditions, including some cancers and type 2 diabetes.
- The general recommendation is for
  - a minimum of 30 minutes a day
  - five days a week
  - exercising to a point of moderate intensity.
- Exercise embraces most movement, including activities that the patient already enjoys.
- Physical activity can be increased at any age and from any level of fitness.

Mental Well-being

- Any cardiovascular disease should be addressed as part of an integrated system which treats the mind, heart, and body as interconnected.
- Robust mental health supports heart health.
- Experiencing a heart attack, other heart event or receiving a heart related diagnosis can have significant psychological implications that should not be ignored.

Scan here for a special free offer for mental well-being insights for a healthier mind-heart connection from James Z G Buckley of the Conscious Mastery Academy.

32	Alicia Philipatos is a blogger and runner. source: https://www.heartfoundation.org.au/Blog/Exercising-for-heart-and-soul
33	further information: www.walking.heartfoundation.org.au
34	Prince SA, et al (2015) Objectively-measured sedentary time and its association with markers of cardiometabolic health and fitness among cardiac rehabilitation graduates. Eur J Prev Cardiol pii: 2047487315617101. [Epub ahead of print]
35	Rogerson M, Le Grande M, Dunstan D et al (2016) Television viewing time and 13-year mortality in adults with cardiovascular disease: Data from the Australian Diabetes, Obesity and Lifestyle Study (AusDiab). Heart Lung Circ. 2017 Nov;26(11):e98-e99. doi: 10.1016/j.hlc.2017.03.153. Epub 2017 Apr 20.
36	Physical activity and your heart health https://www.heartfoundation.org.au/Heart-health-education/physical-activity-and-exercise
37	Among the many references to this is one from the Black Dog Institute https://www.blackdoginstitute.org.au/wp-content/uploads/2020/04/5-exercise_depression.pdf which includes sound, practical advice.
38	Healthline https://www.healthline.com/nutrition/walking-after-eating
39	Robert Zecchin is president of the Australian Cardiovascular Health & Rehabilitation Association (NSW/ACT) and the recipient of the ACRA Alan Goble Distinguished Service Award in 2021. Robert is the Nursing Unit Manager – Cardiac Rehabilitation for Western Sydney Local Health District (WSLHD), and an Adjunct Senior Lecturer, School of Nursing, Faculty of Medicine and Health, University of Sydney. He is a clinician-researcher, has been a collaborator on many multidisciplinary research projects and is a published international author. from an interview with Dr Bishop, podcast # 225 on the Healthy Heart Network, https://drwarrickbishop.com/s/rob
40	Psychological Health, Well-Being, and the Mind-Heart-Body Connection: A Scientific Statement from the American Heart Association; originally published 25 Jan 2021 https://doi.org/10.1161/CIR.0000000000000947 Circulation. 2021;143:e763–e783
41	CIRCULATION https://www.ahajournals.org/doi/10.1161/CIRCULATIONAHA.119.041914 The Mind-Heart-Body Connection, Glenn N. Levine. Originally published 21 Oct 2019 https://doi.org/10.1161/CIRCULATIONAHA.119.041914 Circulation. 2019;140:1363–1365
42	Better Health Channel Heart Disease and Mental Health https://www.betterhealth.vic.gov.au/health/healthyliving/heart-disease-and-mental-health
43	Ralf Ilchef, Healthy Heart Network podcast # 151, https://drwarrickbishop.com/s/ralf, When the heart gets heavy; Warrick Bishop, Alistair Begg, Cardiac Rehabilitation Explained, pp 195-207 (2023)

Obesity is a growing epidemic in the Western World.

chapter 7
OBESITY

> *Refined carbohydrates are incredibly addictive. It is really hard to stop eating those, but it's really important. It's like trying to break a serious addiction ... Help is needed, and it often takes several attempts.*

GEORGIA EDE MD, USA BOARD-CERTIFIED PSYCHIATRIST[44]

Over about the past four decades or so, the incidence of heart attacks gradually declined. This drop was probably related to our better surveillance and better treatment strategies: medications such as aspirin, cholesterol-lowering drugs, blood pressure-lowering drugs, and suitable treatments for heart attacks when they occurred, such as clot-busting medication, devices such as stents for insertion into the arteries and advances in open heart surgery.

However, that trend of decreasing death rates from heart attack changed about 2015, about the time when the incidence of diabetes and obesity reached crisis point. The obesity crisis, a significant concern, is driving us to be more particular about how we think about what we eat and how we move.

undoing the good

The observable First World obesity epidemic is underpinned mainly by the widespread availability of high-caloric, processed, quick, cheap meals. These factors have been disastrous for health, particularly when combined with increased automation and less activity.

A BMI[45] of over 30 presents a significantly increased risk of

- atherosclerotic coronary artery disease – heart attack and stroke,
- cardiac failure, particularly heart failure with preserved function of the heart in which the heart fails to relax well,
- atrial fibrillation, and

- health problems well beyond heart issues, including
  - hypertension (high blood pressure – *see chapter 9*), diabetes (*chapter 10*), sleep apnoea and dementia.

obvious problem

Weight gain is the problem.

A key issue for the patient is the driver behind the weight issue.

- Does the person have an eating disorder?
- Is the person physically inactive or making poor life style choices?

If there is an eating problem, the person needs sound education and, maybe, other professional support. If it's a matter of not having enough physical activity, then

- how much exercise is the person doing
- what type of exercise, and
- how often?

For most people, though, the issue is **what** and **how much** they eat.

The most important thing people can do is be aware of the impact of high-calorie, processed, often sugar-enhanced foods that are easy and quick because of convenience and price. As a society, and individually, we need to recalibrate. It's imperative that we improve our eating, using healthier strategies. For example, we could base our meals on:

- natural foods
- balanced foods
- greens
- meats (and other proteins)
- nuts and fruits (but not too many)

and realise that a healthy, balanced diet with unprocessed food will help reduce the likelihood of progressing to obesity, and pre-diabetes and diabetes *(see chapter 10).*

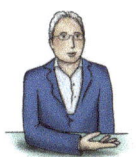

Do not leave check-ups until you see your GP. Instead, take out the tape measure and see for yourself. Waist measurements[46] should be no more than 94 cm for males and 80 cm for females.

complexities

Of course, the challenge is that weight loss becomes complex once the weight is too high.

Although there are many guidelines around this, most focus on caloric restriction. But, of course, there are other considerations, such as socio-economic aspects, mainly financial and psychological impact on the person's life. Therefore, while caloric restriction might be an important basis for discussion, the overall needs, situation and motivation of the individual require consideration.

change

From my clinical experience (WB), several key factors are essential for **achieving** and **sustaining** weight loss.

As many of my patients who have put on excess weight are carbohydrate-sensitive or insulin-resistant, **carbohydrate restriction** is a great starting point. A good clue to carbohydrate sensitivity or insulin resistance is that weight predominantly deposits around the belly, a 'hazardous waist'.

However, even before that, the individual must **want** and be **prepared** to change. That person then should be given information that needs to be turned into knowledge.

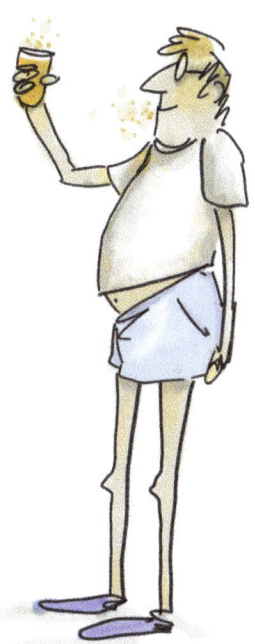

It's essential, too, for patients to have **accountability** – and this is where face-to-face interaction becomes important. Widespread research says face-to-face interaction with someone to support you in losing weight makes the most sense. So, I (WB) generally bring people back for accountability on a two-, three-, or six-monthly basis, depending on how much support I think the person needs.

And lastly, patients may, over and above accountability, need the support that a **coach** can give them:

- if they've done well – rejoice with them, provide lavish approbation,
- if they've done poorly – recognise that life happens. *That's okay; priorities change. Now, let's regroup and start again.*

As well as food intake and type, **exercise and general activity** are significant factors in lifestyle modification to reduce risk. Take the stairs rather than the lift; park further away from you destination and walk the extra distance; have active lunch breaks; incorporate physical activities in hobbies; choose active leisure activities.

Be creative!

If you don't enjoy exercise, you won't do it long-term.

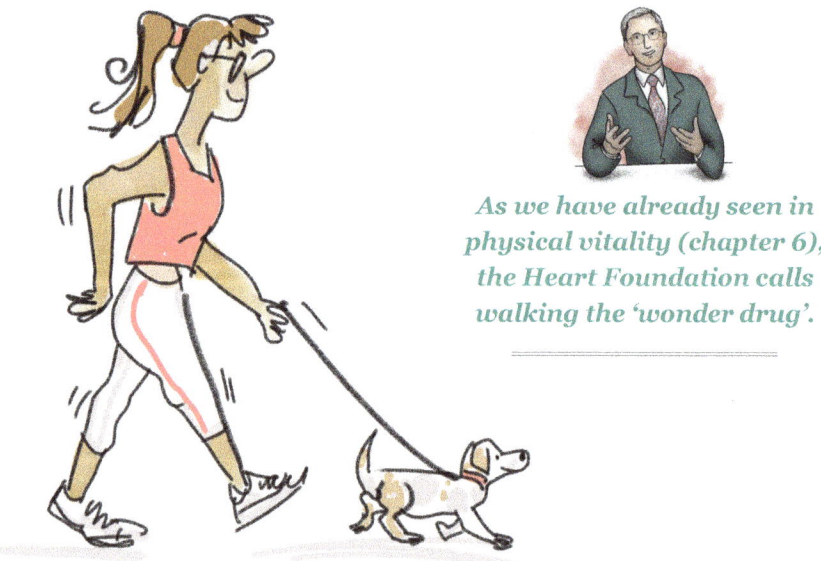

As we have already seen in physical vitality (chapter 6), the Heart Foundation calls walking the 'wonder drug'.

happy, healthy pooch – happy, healthy owner

beyond lifestyle modifications

When a person needs help beyond lifestyle modifications, options exist.

medications

Several drugs are available:

- **liraglutide** and **semaglutide** are GLP-1 agonists[47] that turn off the appetite sensors in the brain. Use of either drug is a great tool to help people miss a meal or begin intermittent fasting. Each also improves metabolism in a way that supports weight loss.
- **duromine** is a stimulant. It drives the sympathetic nervous system, which might raise blood pressure. One should be careful using this with patients prone to high blood pressure or with known CAD.
- **orlistat** is an agent that binds fat within the bowel. It will help reduce the fat calories a person absorbs from the bowel. It 'interferes' with digestive enzymes, limiting fat breakdown in the gut. The undigested fat passes through the gut and is excreted by the bowel.
    - A low-fat diet is essential when taking orlistat or the side effects will prohibit ongoing use.
- the **bupropion-naltrexone** combination is an appetite suppressant that works through the opiate receptors in the brain.

A new, recently released drug for weight loss is **tirzepatide**. Like semaglutide, it is a glucagon-like peptide-1 (GLP-1) receptor agonist. However, it is also a glucose-dependent insulinotropic polypeptide. It works by increasing insulin and decreasing glucagon (a hormone that controls the amount of glucose made by the liver) available in the body. It was developed for the treatment of type 2 diabetes and, like semaglutide, was found to have significant (perhaps greater) weight loss benefits.

surgery

If dietary changes, lifestyle changes and pharmacological therapy do not make much difference, **bariatric surgery** (baro, pressure; iatric, caused by doctor) might be an option. Several alternatives are available *(see following page)*. While bariatric surgery is the last resort, it is a valuable weight loss intervention for the right patient. Long-term results include:

- reduced weight
- reduced blood pressure
- reduced insulin resistance
- improved cholesterol levels
- better sleep
- better quality of life.

Research says that a five per cent or more weight loss benefits individuals in terms of improved blood pressure, cholesterol, and blood sugar levels, as well as an enhanced quality of life.

In Australia, Medicare-funded bariatric facilities – obesity and metabolic clinics – exist but there are waiting times and qualification criteria must be met.

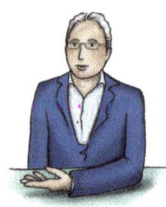

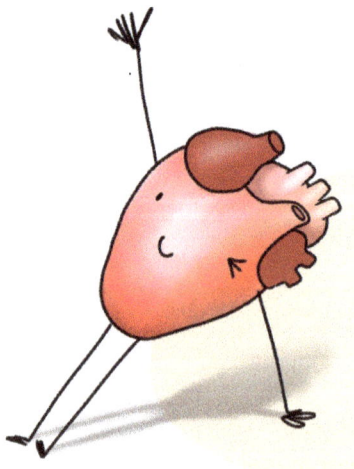

Change is possible, especially:

- with the help of education
- through seeking medical advice
- asking for the support and encouragement of others.

A CLOSER LOOK

bariatric surgery

Bariatric surgery covers a set of weight-loss procedures designed to treat severe obesity when other weight loss methods have been unsuccessful. These surgeries aim to help individuals reduce their food intake, feel fuller faster, and absorb fewer calories from the food they eat. Several types of bariatric surgery are available, with the most common ones being:

1. **gastric bypass (Roux-en-Y)** This procedure involves creating a small pouch at the top of the stomach and bypassing a portion of the small intestine. It restricts the amount of food intake and reduces calorie absorption.

2. **sleeve gastrectomy** A large portion of the stomach is removed, leaving a smaller, banana-shaped stomach. It reduces the capacity for food intake and decreases hunger hormones. This novel surgery is better tolerated with fewer complications than the more traditional gastric band surgery.

3. **adjustable gastric banding** (lap-band) An adjustable band is placed around the upper part of the stomach, creating a small pouch. The band can be tightened or loosened to control food intake.

4. **biliopancreatic diversion with duodenal switch** (BPD/DS) This complex procedure involves a sleeve gastrectomy combined with bypassing a significant portion of the small intestine. It limits food intake and reduces calorie absorption.

Bariatric surgery is typically recommended for individuals with a body mass index (BMI) of 40 or higher, or a BMI of 35-39.9 with obesity-related health conditions such as type 2 diabetes, sleep apnoea, or heart disease.

While bariatric surgery can result in significant weight loss and improve obesity-related health issues, it is not without risks and requires lifelong commitment to dietary and lifestyle changes. It is essential for individuals considering bariatric surgery to undergo a thorough evaluation and discuss the potential risks and benefits with a qualified healthcare professional. Additionally, post-surgery, patients are usually provided with counselling and support to help them adapt to their new eating habits and lifestyle.

IMPORTANT POINTS

OBESITY
- Although this is often a preventable problem, its prevalence is increasing.
- What is the driver behind the weight issue:
  - food choices
  - socio-economic circumstances that lead to the purchase of cheap, poor-quality food
  - lack of education
  - physical inactivity?
- The most common causes are:
  - what a person eats/drinks and
  - how much a person eats/drinks.
- Interventions include:
  - educational programs
  - dietary
  - medication
  - bariatric surgery.
- The patient's GP should be involved in these discussions.

---

44   a USA board-certified psychiatrist, speaking in episode 6, Eating to Prevent Alzheimer's, in the video series Alzheimer's: the Science of Prevention with Dr David Perlmutter (2022)

45   BMI Body Mass Index (adult) is based on the height and weight of a person and is used to determine if a person is in a healthy weight range: < 18.5, underweight; 18.5 to 24.9, healthy weight; 25.0 to 29.9, overweight; 30.0+, obese – 30 to 34.9 obese class I, 35 to 39.9, obese classII, 40+ obese class III (https://www.health.gov.au/topics/overweight-and-obesity/bmi-and-waist)

46   Heart Foundation: https://www.heartfoundation.org.au/Heart-health education/Waistmeasurement

47   GPL-1 is a new class of drugs. The glucagon-like peptide 1 receptor agonists (GLP-1 RAs) act on the incretin hormone system, a system charged with helping the body metabolise carbohydrates. These agents increase glucose-dependent insulin synthesis, suppress appetite, delay gastric emptying and appear to reduce blood pressure, reduce inflammation, and improve vascular endothelial function. (further information: pages 131, 132-133)

Finding a way through the maze of food choices.

chapter 8
'WHAT SHOULD I EAT, DOC?'

One of the most common questions asked of me (WB) is, *What should I eat, Doc.?* And one of the most common things people say to me is, *Well, I have a healthy diet.* What does this mean?

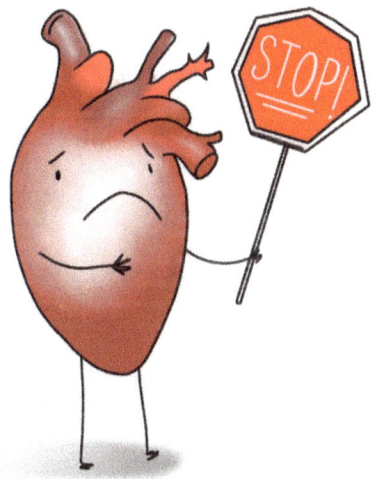

The risk of heart attack implicates diet and lifestyle – of that, there is no question. Nor is there any doubt that **the heart does not enjoy fad diets.**

One of the difficulties with looking at the data concerning nutrition is the trials are challenging to perform and difficult to control. Randomising human beings to very particular diets and managing them is also difficult.

Prospective trials, which start at point zero and **follow** people over time, can be difficult.

Retrospective trials are even less reliable as they ask people to **remember** what they have eaten and what foods they have purchased. These backward-looking trials are often associated with observations of events or occurrences of problems. Another limitation is the inherent inaccuracy of memory.

Retrospective trials do not randomise people but observe one factor and try to link that to an outcome. For example, we might observe in a population that the people who eat the most bananas seem to live the longest. However, that observation in isolation does not tell us the whole picture. Looking further into that observation, we might find that bananas are very, very expensive in that population. So, the only people who can afford to buy bananas are those who can also afford the best health care, giving them the best outcomes.

Although observational data can be fraught with problems, data have been collected on various issues: how much sugar or sodium to have in diets, sugar replacement agents, trans-fats, saturated fats, red meats, processed meats, and the list continues. Even so, this observational and retrospective data can be challenging to interpret.

So, it becomes important for us to focus on prospective studies – those randomised in such a way that they started at a beginning point and followed people through with as much rigour as possible.

The most significant prospective studies provide the best idea of the dietary interventions that are, scientifically, the most validated. The major prospective outcome trials divide into two main groups:

primary prevention

trials that look at preventing people from having the first heart attack or symptoms of heart disease, and

secondary prevention

trials that look at preventing people from having a second heart attack or stopping a second coronary event.

primary prevention

One of the most significant primary prevention trials is the PREDIMED study[48] of 2013.

In a primary prevention study looking at people who had not had a heart attack, the trial took about 7000 Spanish men and women who were at increased risk of heart attack and randomised them to

- a **low-fat** diet
- a **Mediterranean-style** diet enriched with **extra virgin olive oil**
- a **Mediterranean-style** diet supplemented with **nuts**.

The Mediterranean-style diet had more fat than the low-fat diet, was more plant-based, and focused on fish consumption.

The PREDIMED trial strikingly demonstrated an approximately 30 per cent **reduction** in cardiovascular events when the Mediterranean-style diets were eaten compared to the low-fat randomisation. And this was despite the individuals in the Mediterranean diet randomisations having higher LDL ('bad' cholesterol) measurements at the end of the trial.

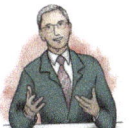

A staggering piece of information! Certainly, a foundation block to the recommendation to use the Mediterranean diet for primary AND secondary prevention of heart disease. Although the article of this study (published by The New England Journal of Medicine*) was retracted in June 2018, a revised look at the updated data produced similar findings*[49] *and was republished.*

secondary prevention

Three main secondary prevention studies are also worth considering:

- Diet and Reinfarction Trial (DART)[50]
- Lyon Diet Heart Study[51]
- The Heart Institute of Spokane Diet and Intervention Trial[52]

DART study

The DART study (conducted about 1990) took more than 2000 men who had suffered a heart attack and randomised them into three diets:

- a **low-fat** diet with an increased ratio of polyunsaturated fats to saturated fats (to try to drive down LDL cholesterol)
- an **omega-3 enriched** diet based on increased fatty fish consumption, and
- a **cereal** or **fibre-based** diet.

The study followed participants over two years.

The outcome was a 30 per cent relative reduction in all-cause mortality in the fatty fish group. This figure is a striking result. But, interestingly, a close examination of those subgroups did not demonstrate a reduction in the reinfarction rate, just a reduction in all-cause mortality.

Lyon Diet Heart Study

The Lyon Diet Heart Study (conducted about 2000) involved about 600 post-heart attack patients, randomised into two different dietary interventions:

- the American Heart Association **low-fat** diet (of the time) and
- a **Mediterranean-style** diet (low in animal products, increased plant-based content, enriched with extra virgin olive oil, while butter and cream were swapped to canola and alpha-linoleic acid).

Over a couple of years, the researchers discovered little difference in the biochemical parameters; the two groups showed little difference in LDL cholesterol. The trial stopped early. During scheduled trial progress evaluation, it became clear that the group on the Mediterranean diet showed a 70 per cent relative risk reduction in non-fatal myocardial infarction (heart attack) and cardiovascular death.

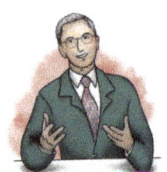

This striking outcome was a big win for good oils, reduced animal products, plant-based eating, and omega-3 oils.

The Heart Institute of Spokane Diet and Intervention Trial

This Spokane study included about 100 patients post heart attack, randomised to

- **usual care**
- a **low-fat** diet or
- a **Mediterranean-style** diet that involved a decrease in saturated fats and an increase in omega-3 oils.

Over the study, there was a clear 30 per cent relative risk reduction in the low-fat **and** Mediterranean dietary intervention groups compared to the usual care group.

what does this mean?

These research data point me (WB) to a clear answer to the question, *What should I eat, Doc.?* regardless of whether the need is primary or secondary prevention. The six key elements of a healthy-living eating pattern are:

1. **plenty** of
    a) whole fruit (not canned or juiced),
    b) vegetables and
    c) whole grains;
2. a variety of **healthy proteins**
    a) especially fish and seafood,
    b) legumes (such as beans and lentils),
    c) nuts and seeds,
    d) a small amount of egg and some poultry, and
    e) if choosing red meat, ensure that the meat is lean, and limit its intake to 1-3 times a week;
3. **dairy** can include
    a) unflavoured milk,
    b) yoghurt, and
    c) cheese;
4. **healthy fat** choices[53] using
    a) nuts,
    b) seeds,
    c) avocados,
    d) olives, and
    e) their oils for cooking[54];
5. **herbs and spices** to flavour the foods instead of adding salt, and
6. the best choice of drink is **water**.

People with high cholesterol and/or diabetes are advised to seek further information and guidance from their health care providers.

An excellent place to start looking for ideas is a Mediterranean-style diet. A healthy-eating plate starts with unprocessed food and consists of one-quarter of protein, one-quarter of carbohydrates, and one-half of vegetables.

top 5 tips

1. **Aim for 5 servings of vegetables a day**. Add vegetables to salads, soups and casseroles or try them as a snack.
2. **Go for grain**. Replace white bread and rice with wholegrain and seeded bread, brown rice, and high-fibre breakfast cereals.
3. **Eat more legumes** such as lentils, chickpeas and beans. Use dried and cooked or canned varieties alone or added to dishes to reduce the amount of meat.
4. **Aim for 2-to-3 servings of oily fish a week.** Canned fish in spring water or olive oil can be used; avoid those canned in brine.
5. Try introducing **at least one meat-free day a week**. You can find lots of quick and tasty meat-free (and other heart-friendly) recipes on the Heart Foundation website (recipes) or visit your country's heart association website.

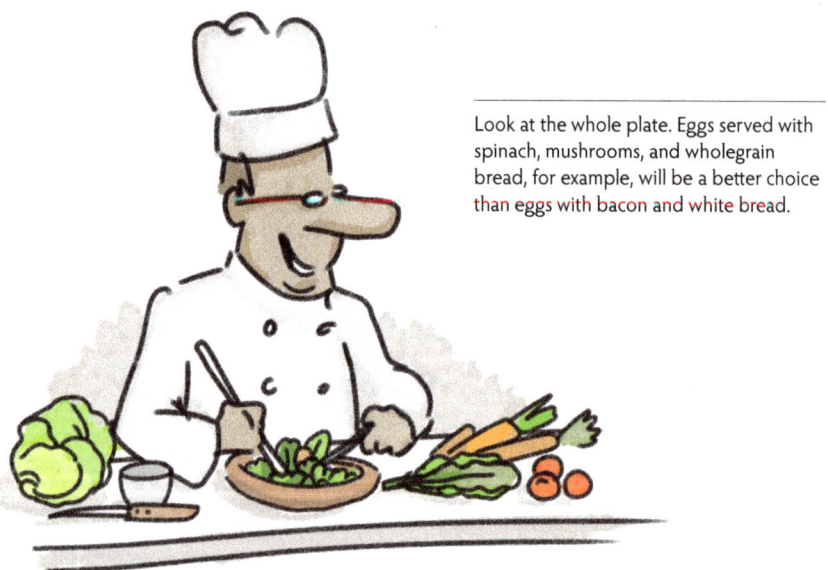

Look at the whole plate. Eggs served with spinach, mushrooms, and wholegrain bread, for example, will be a better choice than eggs with bacon and white bread.

reading food labels

Nutrition information panels and ingredient lists are good ways of comparing similar foods so you can choose the healthiest option. Almost all packaged foods must display a Nutrition Information Panel (NIP) that meets government standards.

The panel is usually on the back or side of the product packaging.

Panels always list:

- energy (kilojoules)
- protein
- fat (total)
- saturated fat
- carbohydrate (total)
- sugars
- sodium.

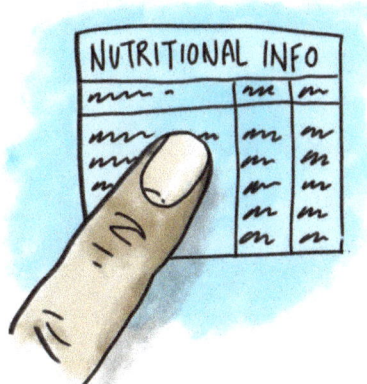

Other nutrients such as vitamins and minerals, fibre and different types of fat may also be listed.

When comparing products, look at the food as a whole rather than deciding based solely on one nutrient. The quantity per 100g or mL column is best when comparing different brands of similar products. Per-serving values vary depending on the type of food and the brand. It doesn't necessarily mean you eat the serving size specified on the pack.

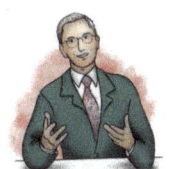

Remember, food that comes unprocessed and without a barcode should always be your first choice.

---

fat Use the 100g or 100mL column to compare similar products to choose the option with less saturated, or trans-fat – the unhealthy fats. Trans-fat is often not listed on the nutrient information panel. Avoid foods with 'partially hydrogenated' vegetable oil or vegetable fat, animal fat, copha and palm oil listed in the ingredients list.

A CLOSER LOOK

please eat more vegies

The (Australian) Heart Foundation wants people to eat more vegetables.[55] Staggeringly, more than 90 per cent of Australians do not eat the recommended five servings of veggies daily. Adding just one serving to a person's daily intake benefits heart health.[56]

If all Australians met the vegetable target, it could cut the risk of cardiovascular diseases by about 16 per cent and save $1.4 billion in health spending.[57]

---

not so simple carbohydrates

Carbohydrates (along with protein and fat) are universal energy sources for our bodies, fuelling our brain, and supporting our overall health. Composed of carbon, hydrogen and oxygen atoms, they come in different forms such as sugars, starches, and fibre. There are two types of carbohydrates: simple and complex. Simple carbohydrates are made up of one or two sugar molecules and are found in foods such as lollies, soft drinks, and baked goods. Complex carbohydrates are made up of many sugar molecules and are found in foods such as whole grains, vegetables, and legumes. When we eat carbohydrates, our body breaks them down into glucose (sugar), which is used as a primary source of energy for our cells.

carbohydrate recommendations

The recommended amount of carbohydrate in the average diet is about 225 to 325 grams of carbohydrates a day, for an 8700 kJ or 2000 calorie diet.

In Australia, the National Health and Medical Research Council set the recommendation for carbohydrates at between 45-65 per cent of total energy intake, which aligns with recommendations from the Institute of Medicine and the World Health Organization, and other leading medical bodies.[58]

salt Salt will show as sodium. Check the ingredient list for other names for salt such as monosodium glutamate and vegetable salt. Use the per 100g column to compare the salt content of two similar products. 'Low salt' means less than 120mg of sodium per 100g of product.

carbs, sugars Simple sugars and complex carbohydrates have the same chemical base – a combination of carbon, hydrogen and oxygen and can be considered a 'hydration of carbon', CH_2O (C for carbon and H_2O for water), a single 'building block' or molecule.

Single or double building blocks are referred to as **simple sugars.** Most people are very familiar with glucose and fructose, which have a single building block structure, and are also called **monosaccharides**. Simple sugars made up of double building blocks are **disaccharides**, such as when glucose and fructose combine and form sucrose (table sugar).

When three or more of these building blocks are strung together, a **complex carbohydrate,** or **polysaccharide,** is formed. Starch and glycogen are two examples.

After consuming carbohydrates – whether they are simple sugars, or complex carbohydrates – they are broken down into their simplest form, monosaccharides, to be used as a source of energy by the body. The main difference lies in how quickly they are digested and absorbed. Simple sugars, typically, are absorbed more rapidly, causing a spike in blood sugar levels, while complex carbohydrates are broken down more slowly, resulting in a more sustained release of glucose into the bloodstream.

When looking at the label, total carbohydrates will include simple sugars, and the proportion of simple sugars to total gives an idea of how much complex carbohydrate or starch is in the food.

More complex and less simple sugars is the way to go.

In my practice (WB), particularly for people seeking to reduce their weight, I advise them to **reduce carbohydrates**. I'm not sure there's a great benefit in large amounts of bread, pasta, rice, potatoes, cereals, fruit and beer for people who want to lose weight or may be at risk of developing diabetes. These foods contain significant amounts of sugar, released as the body digests them.

cook at home

One way to increase fresh produce intake and decrease processed foods is to cook at home more often. Purchased meals and snacks can be high in kilojoules, salt, sugar, and unhealthy fats that are often 'hidden'.

Planning, using leftovers in interesting ways and making your own condiments, including salad dressings and sauces, are also helpful tools.

considerations

Several different components come into play when we consider our eating. Is it to:

- reduce the risk of a heart attack?
- reduce weight?
- reduce the risk of progression to diabetes?

Underpinning each of these considerations is

- a Mediterranean-style diet (as outlined above) that can include eggs in moderation,
- avoid processed foods,
- limit carbohydrates (including complex carbohydrates for weight loss), and
- avoid sugars.

To help you make better choices for your heart health, please visit appendix 3, *swap this for that* (see page 202).

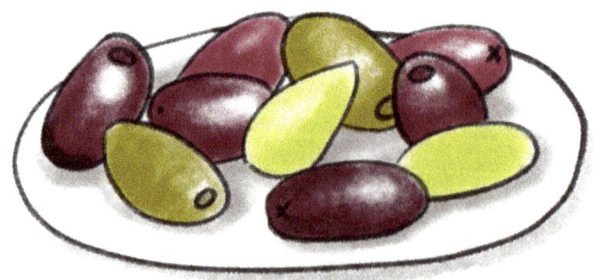

other dietary factors

alcohol

For some time, it has been said that a glass of red might be good for a person's health. This thought is based on the belief that the coloured agents within the 'glass of red', the antioxidants, with some blood pressure lowering and a little HDL raising, could positively impact a person's health.

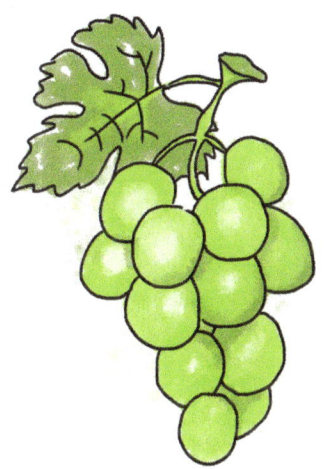

However, the most recent national and international guidelines looking at alcohol have **not** clearly demonstrated any benefit from regular consumption of wine. So, our guidelines from prominent organisations and institutions (2024) have moved away from suggesting that a glass of wine is good for you and now hold a **neutral** position.

The National Health and Medical Research Council's (NHMRC) latest *Australian guidelines to reduce health risks from drinking alcohol*[59] recommends no more than 10 standard drinks[60] per week – with no more than four on any one day – as the maximum for a healthy adult. That amounts to two drinks a day for five days of the week, leaving two days alcohol-free. While you can mix that up any way you like, there is the notion that a day off alcohol each week is a good idea.

Australia's Heart Foundation has an Alcohol Action Plan[61], in electronic and printable forms, designed for people to help manage their alcohol intake. It offers three alternatives within a range of scenarios. For example:

Choose one or two alcohol-free days per week: already doing this / ready to do it now / not yet ready

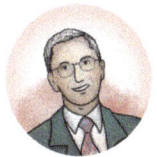

Any lifestyle change is a long and on-going journey. Having a plan makes a huge difference.

THE PLEASURE OF WINE

I believe alcohol has a role beyond health – while sensibly staying within the guidelines already outlined. I think alcohol has become part of our cultural fabric, now having a role in social interaction. As it helps me appreciate a meal, I like half a glass of wine, or even a glass, during the evening, particularly during dinner.

As an aside, well-being is derived from families and friends enjoying meals together. This practice features strongly in the cultures of Mediterranean countries – and is a subtle, and often overlooked, benefit of the Mediterranean diet.[62]

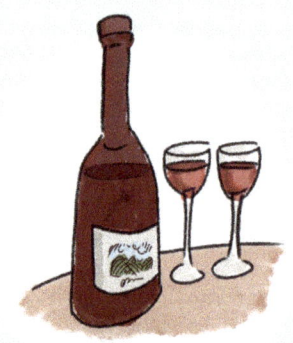

I also enjoy collecting wine. I enjoy going to wineries to purchase a wine that I find interesting, taking it home, laying it down in the cellar, and some years later, sharing it with a friend or family member and, of course, having a story that goes with the wine. Wine, for me, is a passion.

Remember the guidelines: 10 standard drinks per week, with a maximum of four in one session. Please enjoy it – in moderation – along with its socialising connection. And maybe exercise beforehand – a walk to the 'bottle-o' – so you can also benefit from some movement!

As we are stressing throughout this book, education is pivotal to change. A wide range of helpful information is available on any number of trusted websites and from national organisations. Most countries will have their local resources. For several Australian resources, please see footnote 63 at the end of this chapter.

Dr Bishop has a weight loss program:
https://drwarrickbishop.com/s/tfbsg

IMPORTANT POINTS

WHAT SHOULD I EAT, DOC.?

- The heart does not enjoy fad diets.
- Six key elements to a healthy living pattern are:
  - plenty of nuts, whole fruit, vegetables, and whole grains
  - variety of healthy proteins
  - some dairy
  - healthy fat choices
  - herbs and spices
  - water is the drink of choice.
- Five top tips are:
  - aim for 5 servings of vegetables a day
  - go for grain
  - eat more legumes
  - aim for 2-3 servings of oily fish a week
  - aim for at least one meat-free day a week.
- Eat more vegetables.
- Read food labels.
- Cook at home.
- Limit alcohol (but enjoy what you do consume!).

---

48 *Primary Prevention of Cardiovascular Disease with a Mediterranean Diet, April 4, 2013 N Engl J Med 2013; 368:1279-1290 DOI: 10.1056/NEJMoa1200303 https://www.nejm.org/doi/full/10.1056/NEJMoa1200303*

49 *Primary Prevention of Cardiovascular Disease with a Mediterranean Diet Supplemented with Extra-Virgin Olive Oil or Nuts   N Engl J Med 2018; 378:e34 DOI: 10.1056/NEJMoa1800389   https://www.nejm.org/doi/full/10.1056/NEJMoa1800389 PREDIMED trial of Mediterranean diet: retracted, republished BMJ 2019; 364 doi: https://doi.org/10.1136/bmj.l341 (Published 07 February 2019) Cite this as: BMJ 2019;364:l341 https://www.bmj.com/content/364/bmj.l341*

50	https://pubmed.ncbi.nlm.nih.gov/2547617/ DART Clinical Trial Eur Heart J actions Search in PubMed Search in NLM Catalog Add to Search. 1989 Jun;10(6):558-67. doi: 10.1093/oxfordjournals.eurheartj.a059528. Diet and reinfarction trial (DART): design, recruitment, and compliance M L Burr, A M Fehily, S Rogers, E Welsby, S King, S Sandham PMID: 2547617 DOI: 10.1093/oxfordjournals.eurheartj.a059528
51	https://www.ahajournals.org/doi/10.1161/01.cir.103.13.1823 Lyon Diet Heart Study Benefits of a Mediterranean-Style, National Cholesterol Education Program/American Heart Association Step I Dietary Pattern on Cardiovascular Disease Penny Kris-Etherton, Robert H. Eckel, Barbara V. Howard, Sachiko St. Jeor, Terry L. Bazzarre and for the Nutrition Committee Population Science Committee and Clinical Science Committee of the American Heart Association Originally published 3 Apr 2001 https://doi.org/10.1161/01.CIR.103.13.1823 Circulation. 2001;103:1823–1825
52	SPOKANE https://clinicaltrials.gov/ct2/show/NCT00269425
53	Keep away from trans-fats and processed fats.
54	Keep away from vegetable oils.
55	(Australian) Heart Foundation website https://www.heartfoundation.org.au/Bundles/Healthy-Living-and-Eating/Fruit-vegetables-and-heart-health
56	Heart Foundation media release, 8 January 2020; https://www.heartfoundation.org.au/media-releases/what-to-eat-in-2020
57	ibid
58	references include: MedicalNewsToday https://www.medicalnewstoday.com/articles/318617 and NHMRC (National Health and Medical Research Council) https://www.nhmrc.gov.au/ and healthdirect https://www.healthdirect.gov.au/carbohydrates
59	https://www.nhmrc.gov.au/health-advice/alcohol
60	A standard drink contains 10 grams of pure alcohol, regardless of the type of alcohol, and it does not matter if it is mixed with soft drink, fruit juice, water or ice. The (Australian) National Health and Medical Research Council website https://www.nhmrc.gov.au/health-advice/alcohol
61	Heart Foundation website, https://www.heartfoundation.org.au/Heart-health-education/action-plans/alcohol-action-plan. This is one of numerous Action Plans available on the site (https://www.heartfoundation.org.au/Heart-health-education/action-plans/action-plans-index). Although they are offered as recovery after a heart event, they could also be used as lifestyle modification preventative measures.
62	Michael Pollan, In Defence of Food (New York: Penguin Press; 2008)
63	the Heart Foundation (https://www.heartfoundation.org.au/) and in particular pages such as Alcohol and Heart Health: Your Top Questions Answered (dated 22 December 2022) https://www.heartfoundation.org.au/Blog/Alcohol-and-heart-health the Best (and Worst) Drinks for Heart Health – https://www.heartfoundation.org.au/Bundles/Healthy-Living-and-Eating/Heart-healthy-drinks
	the National Alcohol and Other Drug Hotline (https://www.health.gov.au/contacts/national-alcohol-and-other-drug-hotline). Free and confidential advice about alcohol and other drugs is available 24 hours a day, seven days a week on the hotline, 1800 250 015.
	the National Health and Medical Research Council (https://www.nhmrc.gov.au/)

High blood pressure (hypertension) is SO bad for your heart, yet you may not know that you have it!

chapter 9
BLOOD PRESSURE – WHY THE FUSS?

In most first-world countries, hypertension (high blood pressure) is the single most significant modifiable risk factor for plaque build-up or coronary artery disease (*as we described earlier in the book*) – or in medical-speak, atherosclerotic cardiovascular disease (ASCVD), meaning hardening of the arteries. So, high blood pressure is the biggest contributor to heart attack and stroke and a very, very serious global issue. This common problem in modern society affects about a third of adults[64] and often reflects lifestyle choices. It can have a genetic predisposition or sometimes can be from specific medical conditions. More men live with hypertension than women (36.2 per cent to 31.3 per cent, respectively)[65].

Blood pressure is the force of the blood on the artery walls as your heart pumps the blood around your body. It fluctuates throughout the day depending on activity, especially exercise.

Generally, high blood pressure has no specific cause; however, factors can increase a person's chance of developing it, including,

- family history
- eating patterns (including salty foods)
- alcohol intake
- smoking
- weight
- stress
- levels of physical activity.

The prevalence of high blood pressure increases with age.

'**Normal**' adult blood pressure (BP) is said to be a **systolic** BP less than or equal to 130 millimetres of mercury and **diastolic** BP less than or equal to 80 millimetres of mercury, or 130/80 mmHg[66]. For every incremental increase – even one mm of BP – in that systolic or diastolic BP, there is a gradual increase in the risk of heart attack, stroke, and cardiovascular and cerebral vascular consequences. For example, if a person's systolic BP **increased** by 20mm of mercury and the diastolic BP by 10mm, that individual's risk would double. However, even a modest **reduction** in high BP can profoundly affect the risk of heart attack or stroke.

what's the problem?

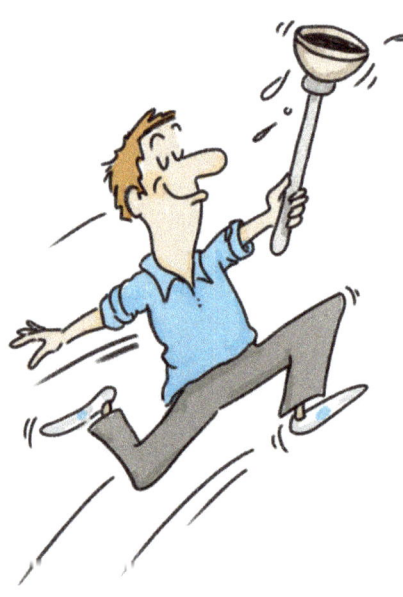

To answer the oft-asked question, *Why is BP so significant?* I (WB) suggest patients imagine they are farmers who have an irrigation system to water the crops.

If the irrigation system pressures can run a bit lower, the **pipes** suffer less wear and tear over the long term. The 'pipes' in the body of most interest to us are the arteries associated with the heart and the brain. The **less wear and tear** on these 'pipes', the **less risk** the person has of a heart attack (heart) or stroke (brain).

A **lower pressure** in the irrigation system **reduces the pressure on the pump**. A pump under pressure can experience a **timing (electrical)** issue. In the body, the heart can respond to prolonged pressure by going into atrial fibrillation (AF), a chaotic and irregular rhythm strongly linked to increased BP.

Sometimes, the system simply **does not work correctly**. As a result, the human pump can develop cardiac failure (CF). In this serious medical condition, the heart becomes stiff and does not relax, and so does not function as it should.

Finally, our irrigation system has a **filtration** system that needs to be kept in good working order as its 'health' impacts the **whole structure**. The body's filtration system is the **kidneys**. So, BP can affect your kidneys – seriously.

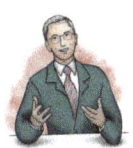 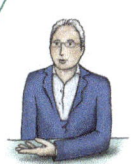

*The 'big four' BP consequences are **heart attack/stroke, atrial fibrillation (AF), cardiac failure (CF), and renal failure**. However, soon it could be the 'big five', as recent evidence also points to an increased risk of **dementia**.*

systolic and diastolic

To better understand BP, we need to understand systolic and diastolic BP.

Systolic BP relates to the highest BP in the vascular tree and coincides with the **heart's contraction when the aortic valve is open** and blood is being 'squeezed' from the heart's left ventricle (its main pumping chamber) into the aorta (the beginning of the vascular tree). **Systole** is the term used for the **contraction** of the heart.

Diastolic BP is measured when the **aortic valve is closed**. When the heart finishes contracting, it relaxes, the pressure drops, and the aortic valve closes. **Diastole** is the term used for the **relaxation** of the heart. Because the aortic valve is closed, the inside of the heart and the vasculature (the blood vessels) are not connected. Therefore, when the heart squeezes, the measured pressure directly relates to how hard the heart is squeezing.

Imagine this. We are trying to measure systolic BP. The heart squeezes very vigorously. The aorta and other large arteries distend (or stretch) complying with the increased force, absorbing much of that energy; the pressure may not be very high. However, if the heart squeezes with the same vigour but the arteries cannot distend because they are stiff, the force from the heart contracting is transmitted to the vascular system, pushing up the blood pressure.

When the heart has finished contracting, the recoil of the large blood vessels, such as the aorta, determines the diastolic BP. Think again of the heart squeezing hard and the aorta stretching (dilating). When the heart stops contracting, it 'springs' back, yielding energy, which is the diastolic BP. When the heart stops contracting and the aortic valve closes, if the aorta is stiff, there is not much recoil; there is not a lot of energy to maintain the diastolic BP, and it is relatively low.

Commonly seen hypertension in the elderly best demonstrates this process. As a person's arteries (including the aorta) stiffen, the systolic BP goes up because not much energy is absorbed effectively by the aortic wall, and the diastolic pressure drops. This big gap left between the systolic and diastolic pressures is known as **isolated systolic hypertension**, a common form of BP in people older than 65 years of age.

measurements

How is BP measured? Traditionally, it has been determined in the doctor's office using a **cuff wrapped around the patient's arm**. That method is subject to variability, not least of which is the anxiety level being experienced by the patient at the time of the measurement. And in 20 to 25 per cent of people, their BP goes up regardless – and that's called 'white coat' hypertension (from the days when doctors wore white coats!).

A common practice now is for people to measure their BP at **home** numerous times, thus mitigating any perceived stress from being in a doctor's office. Using the correct cuff size is essential, as is sitting quietly for a few minutes before taking the measurement.

Another measurement method is use of a **24-hour BP monitor**. A BP cuff stays on the patient for 24 hours, measuring the BP every 30 minutes during the day and every hour overnight. The result is a beautiful profile of what's going on with the individual's BP.

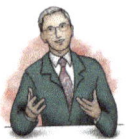
For me (WB), the 24-hour BP monitor is the current (2024) clinical gold standard and my preferred way of checking BP.

A **catheter in an artery** can also be used to measure BP. This method, which obtains precise information, is employed in intensive care units, cardiac cath. labs and sometimes during complex surgeries, rather than in clinical outpatient settings. Such readings inform medicos about the accuracy of other modalities used for measuring BP.

New technologies are attempting to sample the artery, the artery wall, and the pulse pressures in different ways. As a result, the coming years will undoubtedly provide the medical profession with innovative opportunities for detecting BP more effectively – probably at home, and probably in association with smartphones and apps.

treatment

Before treatment starts, a definite diagnosis involving accurate measurements is needed.

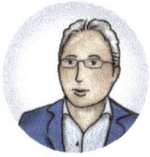

There should be no guesswork here![67]

Once tests establish elevated BP, lifestyle measures, especially weight loss, salt restriction, and exercise, are excellent starting points to reduce the level.

Eat a healthy diet (less salt, less sugar, less 'bad' fats and more 'healthy' fats). If a patient is overweight, one kilogram of weight loss is associated with one millimetre of BP reduction. So, losing five to 10 kilograms is about as effective as giving someone a tablet. Interestingly, dark chocolate, in moderation, can reduce BP and it also contains beneficial antioxidants.

Be physically active. Exercise can lower BP. Regular exercise, two to four times a week (with some wriggle), can lower BP by about five millimetres of mercury. This, again, is nearly as effective as a single medication.

Other lifestyle factors involve managing blood cholesterol levels and diabetes. Do not smoke. Limit alcohol consumption, as excessive alcohol consumption links strongly to elevated blood pressure.

Look after one's **mental health**.

Medications and **medical procedures** are available.

ANSWERING YOUR QUESTIONS

is there a 'perfect' BP?

Let's start to answer the question, *Is there a 'perfect' BP?* by considering BP as a low-to-high continuum.

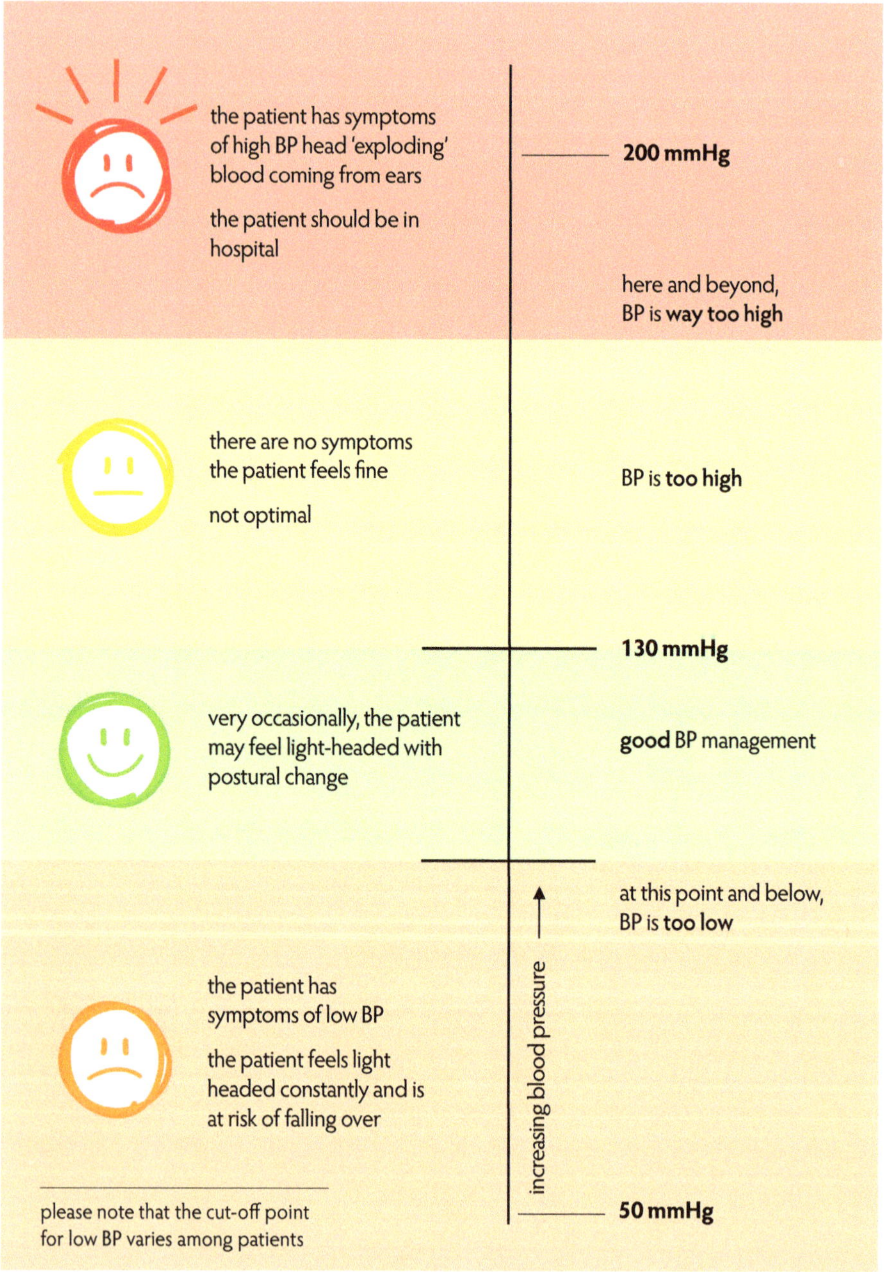

	the patient has symptoms of high BP head 'exploding' blood coming from ears	**200 mmHg**
	the patient should be in hospital	here and beyond, BP is **way too high**
	there are no symptoms the patient feels fine	BP is **too high**
	not optimal	
		130 mmHg
	very occasionally, the patient may feel light-headed with postural change	**good** BP management
		at this point and below, BP is **too low**
	the patient has symptoms of low BP the patient feels light headed constantly and is at risk of falling over	
please note that the cut-off point for low BP varies among patients		**50 mmHg**

↑ increasing blood pressure

When they were 10 years old, our children would have had low blood pressures compared to our elderly parents, whose BPs would have been relatively high. For most of our patients – particularly those at high risk of, say, a heart attack or developing CF or AF – we want to be precise in their BP level.

So, recognising this BP continuum, we try to find the lowest point we can get their BP to without them developing ongoing symptoms from their BP being too low.

This is represented on the diagram (*previous page*) by the black line between the green and orange colours. We haven't included a specific number here because this figure changes for each patient.

The symptoms of low BP include light-headedness – from activities such as standing up, bending over, or getting out of bed – associated with loss of energy. We don't want people to live like that. Still, we attempt to get them very close to that switching point.

Patients might experience some light-headedness once or twice a week, which they will understand is because of their tablets. Then, we've got them as low as possible, with negligible side effects while receiving genuine benefit from keeping their BP down. If they're above that point and not experiencing any symptoms, we can't be sure we have them as low as possible.

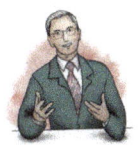
Controlling blood pressure is not as sexy or exciting as riding in the back of an ambulance or having a stent inserted into an artery. Still, it is the single most helpful intervention for long-term cardiovascular health.
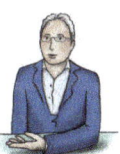

medications

Fortunately, well trialled, and effective blood pressure therapies are available. These agents work through different modalities within the body and, so, some suit some patients better than others. Often, there can be a process of trial and error to identify the best match for an individual patient. Commonly used anti-hypertensive drugs include:

- **angiotensin-converting enzyme (ACE) inhibitors** work by blocking the conversion of angiotensin I to angiotensin II, a hormone that narrows blood vessels and raises blood pressure. By doing so, they help relax blood vessels and lower blood pressure.
    - examples include enalapril, lisinopril, and ramipril;
- **angiotensin II receptor blockers (ARBs)** block the action of angiotensin II at its receptors, similar to ACE inhibitors, resulting in vasodilation and reduced blood pressure.
    - examples include losartan, valsartan, and candesartan;
- **calcium channel blockers (CCBs)** inhibit the entry of calcium into muscle cells of the heart and blood vessels, leading to relaxation and widening of blood vessels. This helps reduce blood pressure.
    - examples include amlodipine, nifedipine, and diltiazem;
- **diuretics**, often referred to as 'water pills', increase the excretion of sodium and water from the body, reducing the volume of blood and subsequently lowering blood pressure.
    - examples include hydrochlorothiazide and furosemide;
- **beta-blockers** prevent the effects of adrenaline and other stress hormones on the heart, leading to a decrease in heart rate and a reduction in the force of heart contractions. this results in lowered blood pressure.
    - examples include metoprolol, atenolol, and propranolol;
- **centrally-acting antihypertensive agents** work on the central nervous system to reduce blood pressure. By targeting specific receptors in the brain, they decrease the sympathetic nervous system's activity, which leads to reduced signals for vasoconstriction (narrowing of blood vessels) and a subsequent decrease in blood pressure.
    - examples include clonidine, methyldopa, and moxonidine;

- **vasodilators** work by dilating (widening) the blood vessels, which leads to a reduction in blood pressure. By relaxing the smooth muscles in the walls of arteries and veins, vasodilators increase the diameter of blood vessels, allowing blood to flow more easily and with less resistance. This results in decreased pressure on the arterial walls. They can be used as standalone drugs for hypertension or may be prescribed in combination with other antihypertensive medications.
  - examples include: hydralazine, minoxidil (typically reserved for cases of severe or resistant hypertension due to potential side effects), sodium nitroprusside (for fast-acting intravenous use in hypertensive emergencies), nitro-glycerine (primarily used to relieve angina), and alpha-blockers (often used in combination with other drugs) this direct-acting vasodilator relaxes the smooth muscles of the arterioles, leading to reduced peripheral resistance and lowering of blood pressure.

The choice of drug or combination of drugs depends on factors such as the patient's overall health, medical conditions, and potential side effects. Your doctor will work with you to find your therapeutic best fit.

procedures

Research is evolving a procedure to facilitate management of blood pressure control, particularly for people who respond poorly to medications.

This procedure, **renal artery denervation**, works on the premise that the nerves of the sympathetic nervous system (the 'fight and flight' system) that run along the renal artery to the kidneys play an important role in driving elevated blood pressure through kidney mechanisms. When over-active, they contribute to high blood pressure.

Renal artery denervation uses a catheter (a specialised tube) passed through an artery in the leg to place a specialised device in the renal artery. This device uses radio frequency (destructive energy) to ablate or destroy the nerves running along the outside of the renal artery to the kidney.

This procedure has been in and out of favour over the years. However, recent studies show promising results, so we may see more of this procedure soon, particularly for those patients with difficult-to-control pressures.

IMPORTANT POINTS

BLOOD PRESSURE – WHY THE FUSS?

- A modest reduction in high blood pressure can have a profound effect on the risk of heart attack or stroke.
- Lifestyle modifications can help to control blood pressure.
- Medications and medical procedures can be used.
- Accurate blood pressure readings are essential before starting treatment and in assessing response to treatment.
- Achieving and maintaining good BP is high on the list of cardiac prevention measures.

---

64 Heart Foundation: https://www.heartfoundation.org.au/Activities-finding-or-opinion/key-statistics-risk-factors-for-heart-disease

65 ibid.

66 In Australia, Heart Foundation website, https://www.heartfoundation.org.au/Heart-health-education/Blood-pressure-and-your-heart. However, a doctor will advise the patient based on medical history and other circumstances.

67 The European guidelines say that the 24-hour blood pressure monitoring should be done before initiating any blood pressure treatment, to confirm the patient does have high blood pressure. 2020 International Society of Hypertension Global Hypertension Practice Guidelines Thomas Unger et al. originally published 6 May 2020 https://doi.org/10.1161/HYPERTENSIONAHA.120.15026 Hypertension. 2020; 75:1334–1357

When sugar is not so sweet.

chapter 10
BLOOD SUGAR OVERLOAD

 Sugar has been found to be as addictive as cocaine.

GEORGIA EDE MD, USA BOARD-CERTIFIED PSYCHIATRIST[68]

In both pre-type 2 diabetes and type 2 diabetes, blood sugar and insulin levels are higher than normal.

Put simply, pre-diabetes occurs when the blood sugar level is higher than normal, yet it is not high enough to be considered type 2 diabetes. A type 2 diabetes diagnosis occurs when the fasting blood sugar level is greater than 7.0 mmol/l or when the haemoglobinA1c (HbA1c) – a marker for sugar-affected protein in the blood – is greater than 6.5 per cent.

Diabetes is not one condition. About 10 to 15 per cent of the population of major western economies has one of two types[69] of diabetes[70]:

- **type 1 diabetes** (characterised by **inadequate** or negligible insulin production) – juvenile-onset diabetes, in which there is an auto-immune problem with the pancreas, and it stops producing insulin. These sufferers need to inject insulin, often from a young age; and
- **type 2 diabetes** (characterised initially by **increased** or excessive insulin production) – in which individuals tend to progress from obesity to insulin resistance to pre-diabetes, then to raised blood sugars and diabetes. This group embraces 90 to 95 per cent of all people with diabetes.

what is type 2 diabetes?

Diabetes occurs when there is a loss of the finely tuned balance between insulin production in the pancreas and tissue response to insulin. As a consequence, the person's blood sugar levels rise. To understand this better, we must first look more closely at the naturally occurring insulin.

insulin

Insulin is a storage hormone, produced by the pancreas that regulates the amount of glucose in the blood (blood sugars). Glucose is the body's primary source of energy and is essential for the brain. It comes from 'complex' carbohydrates (food such as bread, cereals, fruit, starchy vegetables, sweets) being broken down to 'simple' sugars. When this glucose enters the blood stream, the pancreas secretes insulin, which allows the glucose to enter the body's cells to generate energy. Because glucose levels are high after eating, surplus glucose is stored in the liver as glycogen, to be released into the blood stream between meals when the glucose levels are low. This mechanism maintains the body's blood sugar levels within a narrow and balanced range.

diabetes

After eating, individuals with diabetes, experience persistently elevated glucose levels due to insulin's inability to move the glucose into the cells. Those with type 2 diabetes do not utilise insulin sufficiently (insulin resistance). They may produce excess insulin, but it may not be adequate to control blood sugar levels (relative insulin deficiency). Individuals with type 1 diabetes, on the other hand, produce little or no insulin.

no discrimination

Anyone can develop diabetes. Type 2 can be hereditary, although it is often directly related to lifestyle choices mainly associated with obesity and a sedentary routine. Hypertension (high blood pressure) and abnormal blood lipids (high cholesterol) also contribute significantly.

In type 2 diabetes, many people have no symptoms. Signs can go unnoticed or be seen as part of 'getting older'. Therefore, complications may already be present when the person notices problems. Common symptoms[71] include:

- being more thirsty than usual
- passing more urine

- feeling tired and lethargic
- always feeling hungry
- having cuts that heal slowly
- itchy skin infections
- blurred vision
- unexplained weight loss (type 1)
- gradual increase in weight (type 2)
- mood swings
- headaches
- feeling dizzy
- leg cramps.

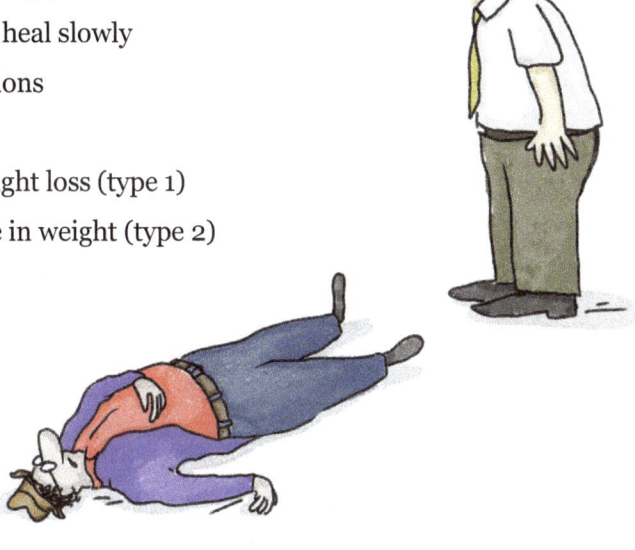

serious

Diabetes is a serious and complex condition that can affect the entire body.

People with type 2 diabetes are two to four times more likely to develop cardiovascular diseases (CVD), such as heart attack and stroke. CVD is the leading cause of mortality for people with type 2 diabetes[72]. The potential for damaged nerves and blood vessels also opens the person to the possibility of a 'silent' heart attack, which lacks the typical chest pain.

According to Diabetes Australia[73], diabetes:

- is the leading cause of blindness in working-age adults;
- is a leading cause of kidney failure and the need for dialysis;
- increases the risk of heart attacks and stroke by up to four times;
- is a major cause of limb amputations, and
- affects mental and physical health – depression, anxiety, and distress occur in more than 30 per cent of all people with diabetes.

no simple cure

Diabetes has **no simple cure**, but it can be **managed**[74] and, if caught early enough, **reversed**.

Diabetes adds **complexity** to the cardiovascular scene. People with diabetes do not respond well to standard treatments, and the outcomes are worse than for people who do not have diabetes. Therefore, prevention and management need good control of dietary intake, particularly sugars, as well as attention to exercise, weight control and, where indicated, medications. *(Please re-read the relevant chapters.)*

A decrease in atherosclerotic cardiovascular disease (ASCVD) rates among people with diabetes has been noted in recent years. This drop is testimony to the enormous input into primary prevention in this group by

- treating elevated blood pressure,
- gaining control over raised sugar levels with improving agents, and
- prudent management of cholesterol levels using statins.

Even with such positive advancements, ASCVD remains the main cause of mortality and morbidity for people with diabetes.

stay healthy – manage weight

The overarching issue is to **avoid that initial weight gain**. Maintain a healthy weight. Losing one, two, or five kilograms is much easier than undergoing a 15 or 20-kilo-weight-loss journey.

However, if excessive weight is the diabetic driver, a large weight loss can reverse type 2 diabetes.

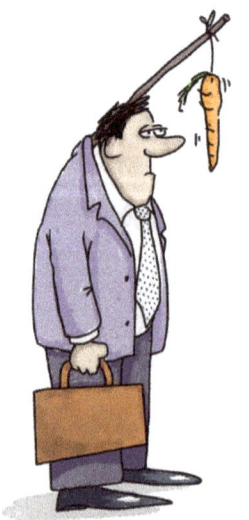

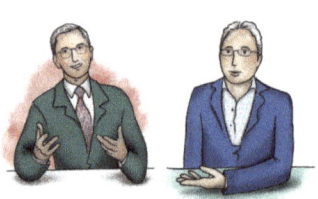

Our strong advocacy is: Always keep a close eye on your weight. If it is creeping up, take action to start it moving down. Early intervention is much, much better for many reasons than leaving it too late.

medications

Several medications are available to help manage diabetes type 2. They include:

- **metformin** which is widely prescribed as the first-line medication for type 2 diabetes. It helps lower blood sugar levels by improving insulin sensitivity and reducing glucose production by the liver;
- **sulfonylureas** stimulate the pancreas to produce more insulin, helping to lower blood sugar levels. They are often used when metformin alone is insufficient to control blood glucose levels.
    - examples, gliclazide, glimepiride;
- **dipeptidyl peptidase-4** (DPP-4) **inhibitors** work by increasing insulin production and reducing the liver's glucose output. They also help lower blood sugar levels after meals by slowing down the breakdown of incretin hormones.
    - examples, sitagliptin, linagliptin;
- **sodium-glucose transporter 2** (SGLT2) **inhibitors** work by blocking the reabsorption of glucose by the kidneys, leading to increased glucose excretion in the urine and helping to lower blood sugar levels.
    - examples, empagliflozin, dapagliflozin;
- **glucagon-like peptide 1** (GLP-1) **receptor agonists** stimulate the release of insulin and suppress glucagon secretion, both of which lower blood sugar levels. They also slow down gastric emptying and help with weight loss.
    - examples, liraglutide, exenatide.

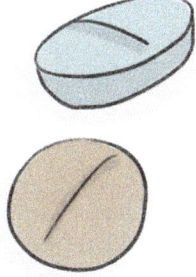

A CLOSER LOOK

new drugs - sodium-glucose co-transporter 2 inhibitors

Very recently, one of the most exciting advances for making a difference for people who have diabetes and cardiac failure is with a group of drugs called gliflozins or sodium-glucose transport inhibitors (SGLT2 inhibitors). Initially, research interest focussed on one in particular, empagliflozin (as others were becoming available).

The EMPA-REG trial[75], which looked at empagliflozin, and was designed principally for diabetes management, showed (much to the investigators' surprise) an impressive reduction in cardiac failure complications in the treatment group. As we have already seen, diabetes complicates the cardiac scenario.

Gliflozin agents work at the kidney's proximal tubule, shutting down sodium-glucose transport. This action means that sodium and glucose filtered out of the blood by the kidneys are not reabsorbed into the blood, allowing the loss of salt and sugar into the urine. (Retained salt leads to retained fluid which leads to elevated blood pressure. Not good!)

Lower blood glucose levels mean less sugar in the body, thus benefitting sugar levels and weight loss.

The use of SGLT2 inhibitors has shown a clear benefit in the reduction of mortality and reduction of hospitalisations with improved quality of life for diabetic patients with cardiac failure.

The gliflozins are under extensive investigation. Agents now include canagliflozin, dapagliflozin, empagliflozin and ertugliflozin.

Thrush is the most common side effect. Care needs to be taken to monitor renal function. Stopping the agents before surgery is recommended.

glucagon-like peptide 1 receptor agonists

Another new class, GLP-1 drugs – the glucagon-like peptide 1 receptor agonists (GLP-1 RAs) – acts on the incretin hormone system, a system charged with helping the body metabolise carbohydrates. These agents increase glucose-dependent insulin synthesis (meaning that for a given exposure of glucose, the body produces more insulin), suppress appetite (through the central nervous system), delay gastric emptying and appear to reduce blood pressure and inflammation, and improve vascular endothelial function.

This class of agents improves not only diabetic control but also aids in weight loss and, so, control of high blood pressure – all of which are good for the heart.

GLP-1 RA drugs include semaglutide and dulaglutide – both have the convenience of once-weekly dosage – and exenatide, which is taken twice daily. These agents tend to result in better blood sugar control than the SGLT2 agents and are the preferred add-on to metformin unless the patient has cardiac or renal failure where the SGLT2 agents have shown clear benefits.

Patients generally tolerate these drugs well. Gastrointestinal issues are the main reported side effect.

The benefits of reduced appetite and weight loss can't be underestimated in this group of patients.

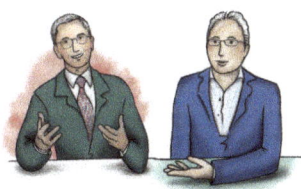

This space of diabetic medications that have a role in reducing cardiovascular risk or cardiac-related outcomes is an exciting one and is currently (2024) advancing in leaps and bounds.

IMPORTANT POINTS

BLOOD SUGAR OVERLOAD

- Diabetes adds complexity to heart conditions.
- Prevention is the key, especially if the person is
  - overweight
  - makes poor dietary choices
  - leads a sedentary lifestyle.
- A new class of drugs (sodium-glucose transporter inhibitors, SGLT 2 inhibitors) for diabetes is proving helpful for cardiac patients who suffer cardiac failure or who experience blood pressure and weight issues.
- Another new class of drugs (glucagon-like peptide 1 receptor agonists, GLP-1 RAs) also improves diabetic management and supports weight loss and control of high blood pressure.

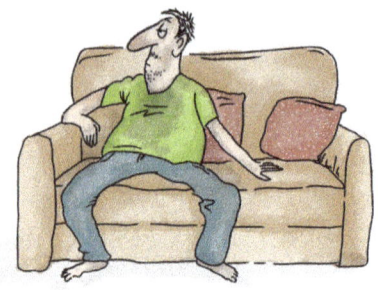

68 Speaking in episode 6, Eating to Prevent Alzheimer's, in the video series Alzheimer's: the Science of Prevention with Dr David Perlmutter (2022)

69 Alzheimer's disease sometimes is referred to as 'type 3 diabetes' because some scientists believe that insulin dysregulation in the brain causes dementia. However, type 3 diabetes is not an officially recognised health condition. (2022)

70 There is also gestational diabetes (GDM) that occurs during pregnancy. This is the fastest growing type of diabetes in Australia and usually occurs around the 24th to 28th week of pregnancy. Diabetes Australia, https://www.diabetesaustralia.com.au/about-diabetes/gestational-diabetes/

71 This information on diabetes comes from the diabetes Australia website with the note that this information is of a general nature only and should not be substituted for medical advice or used to alter medical therapy. It does not replace consultations with qualified healthcare professionals to meet individual medical needs.
https://www.diabetesaustralia.com.au/about-diabetes/what-is-diabetes/

72 Heart Foundation, https://www.heartfoundation.org.au/Heart-health-education/Diabetes-and-heart-disease

73 Diabetes Australia, https://www.diabetesaustralia.com.au/about-diabetes/what-is-diabetes/

74 ibid.

75 Empagliflozin, Cardiovascular Outcomes, and Mortality in Type 2 Diabetes
Authors, Bernard Zinman, M.D. et al, and Silvio E. Inzucchi, M.D. for the EMPA-REG OUTCOME Investigators November 26, 2015 N Engl J Med 2015; 373:2117-2128
DOI:10.1056/NEJMoa1504720
https://www.nejm.org/doi/full/10.1056/NEJMoa1504720
conclusions: Patients with Type 2 diabetes at high risk for cardiovascular events who received empagliflozin, as compared with placebo, had a lower rate of the primary composite cardiovascular outcome and of death from any cause when the study drug was added to standard care.
editorial: Cardiovascular Risk and Sodium–Glucose Cotransporter 2 Inhibition in Type 2 Diabetes, Julie R. Ingelfinger, M.D., Clifford J. Rosen, M.D. November 26, 2015 N Engl J Med 2015; 373:2178-2179 DOI: 10.1056/NEJMe1512602 https://www.nejm.org/doi/full/10.1056/NEJMe1512602?query=recirc_curatedRelated_article

It helps to be ahead of the game.

chapter 11
SHOULD WE GUESS OR TAKE A LOOK?

As we already know, most risk factors are modifiable and linked to a person's lifestyle; some are not, including age, gender, ethnicity, and family history.

non-modifiable risks

Simply getting **older** is a heart disease risk factor.

Men have a greater risk of heart disease than women. However, after menopause, a woman's risk starts approaching that of a man's, and the outcomes worsen.

People with African, Asian, or Aboriginal and Torres Strait Islander **ancestry** are at higher risk than other ethnic groups.

The risk of cardiovascular disease associated with **family** and genes focuses on **early onset** in siblings and parents (referred to as 'first degree' relatives) rather than a 93-year-old great uncle. Early onset generally means having suffered CVD before the age of 55 for men and 60 for women. Often genetically high cholesterol, a condition called **familial hypercholesterolemia**, causes early onset.

If both parents have suffered heart disease before turning 55, a person's risk of developing heart disease can rise to 50 per cent compared to the general population. This heightened risk is particularly so if there are other significant contributing issues such as a history of smoking, raised cholesterol, marked obesity, pre-diabetes or type 2 diabetes.

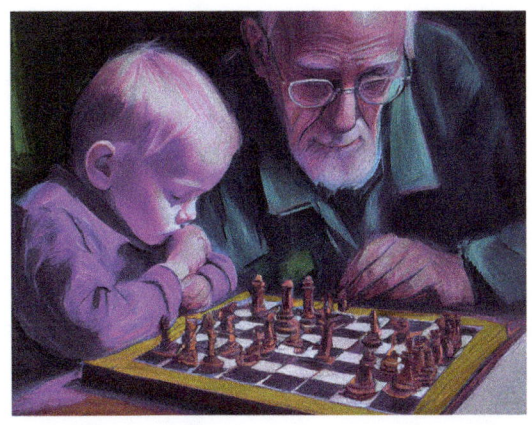

moving forward

After a coronary artery event or a CAD diagnosis, the way forward is very clear: re-establish or improve the blood flow and implement secondary prevention strategies to reduce the risk of repetition or further deterioration of the condition. As we have already seen, methods used include medication, lowering cholesterol levels and lifestyle modifications.

However, the situation is not as clear-cut when it involves patients who have **not** had a problem. They do not display any symptoms, nor have they been defined yet as having a problem. Still, they might be at high risk because of indicators such as cholesterol levels, high blood pressure, diabetes, or smoking.

The treatment for that risk – before an event – is **primary prevention**, aimed at stopping a primary or first event.

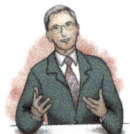

You have heard of 'fit and well' individuals suffering a heart attack 'out of the blue' to everyone's surprise. Just bad luck! Or is it?

I (WB) believe that aspects of our current approach to primary prevention have significant limitations, for example, using the stress test as an indicator of coronary artery disease risk in an asymptomatic person..

The **exercise stress test**, usually undertaken on a treadmill or a stationary exercise bike, determines **how blood flows through the arteries**. By recalling our earlier discussion about flow-limiting and non-flow-limiting plaque *(see pages 46-47)*, you will appreciate that this testing has a limitation.

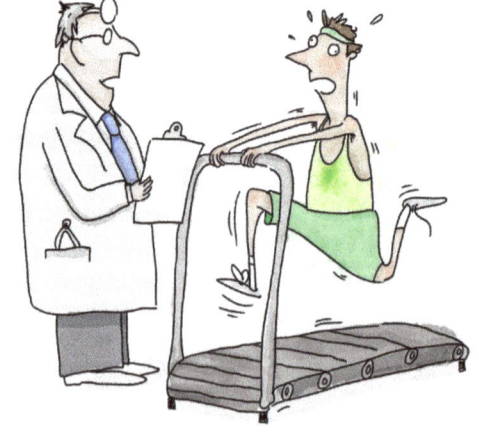

A significant amount of **plaque** can build up in the arteries **before** it leads to a narrowing and, therefore, **before** it shows any features on stress testing. Thus, it is **late** in the process when it is detected as a problem.

To a degree, that patient has run the gauntlet of a major event with potential rupture of the non-flow-limiting plaque, which would remain undetectable because it causes no limitation to flow until the moment it ruptures, forms a clot, and blocks the artery.

patient 'pictures'

A picture paints 1000 words.

One of the key tools in our primary prevention approach is to use the latest technology available to **scan the heart**.

By scanning the heart, we can obtain as much information as possible about the condition of the arteries of the patient's heart by looking at the arteries to see what is happening.

The case studies that follow are patients of Dr Bishop.

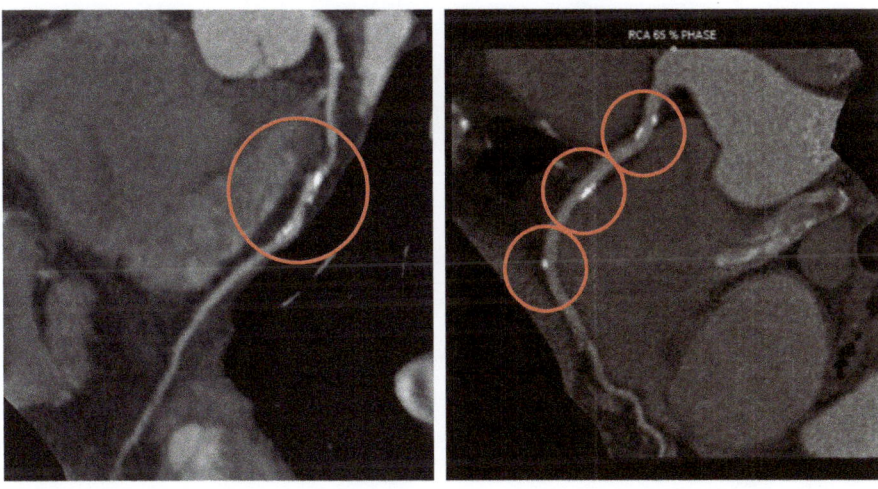

These are images from a cardiac CT scan done on a 61-year-old fireman who had had a 'normal' exercise stress test, exercising for 12 minutes without problems. He still wanted more reassurance as he had a history of high blood pressure, and there was a family history of coronary disease and diabetes. The scans clearly show a significant build-up of plaque that could not be picked up by the stress testing. This additional information allowed for appropriate risk management that otherwise would not have been undertaken.

PATIENT'S PERSPECTIVE – CONRAD

I have had moderately high cholesterol levels for the past 30 years and have it checked annually by my GP. Given this history, I recently sought advice from my GP regarding a test I could have to identify any early signs of heart disease. My GP recommended Dr Warrick Bishop as he specialises in the early detection and prevention of heart disease. This approach is precisely what I was seeking.

Based on my history and lifestyle, Dr Bishop indicated that my risk of heart disease would be at the lower end of the scale, but, to provide further peace of mind for the next five to 10 years, I could have a cardiac CT scan. Dr Bishop clearly explained the minimal risks associated with the procedure.

In lay terms, he described how the CT scan takes a series of individual x-rays that combine to make a 3D picture of the heart and arteries. Such 3D images show any build-up of plaque in the artery walls. Dr Bishop advised me upfront that Medicare did not cover this procedure. However, the resulting peace of mind far outweighed the modest cost.

The CT scan was straightforward and took only a few minutes plus 30 minutes of monitoring before and after. My appointment started at 9 am, and I was back at work before 10 am. The procedure's worst part was that I did not have my usual cup of coffee first thing in the morning!

I would not hesitate to have a cardiac CT scan in the future.

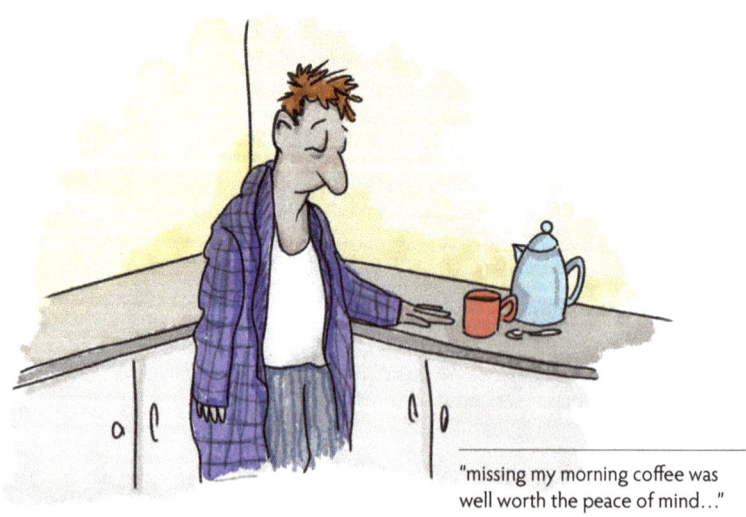

"missing my morning coffee was well worth the peace of mind…"

PATIENT PICTURES – TRACEY AND BECK   CASE STUDY

Two sisters, Tracey and Beck, came to see me. Both had elevated cholesterol levels and a family history of premature coronary artery disease. They were in their early 50s, and neither wanted to take cholesterol-lowering medication unless necessary.

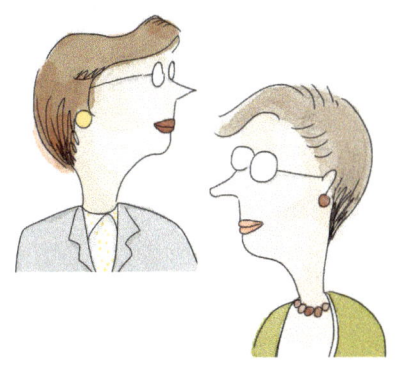

Their lipid profiles were:

Tracey

Total Cholesterol (TC)	8.2	ideally < (less than) 5.0 mmol/l
Triglycerides (TG)	2.2	ideally <2.0 mmol/l
High Density Lipoprotein (HDL)	1.0	ideally > (greater than) 1.0 mmol/l
TC to HDL ratio	8.2	ideally <4.0 ratio
Non HDL	7.2	ideally <4.0 mmol/l
Low Density Lipoprotein (LDL)	6.2	ideally <2.5 mmol/l*

Beck

Total Cholesterol (TC)	10.6	ideally < (less than) 5.0 mmol/l
Triglycerides (TG)	12.5	ideally <2.0 mmol/l
High Density Lipoprotein (HDL)	0.8	ideally > (greater than) 1.0 mmol/l
TC to HDL ratio	13.3	ideally <4.0 ratio
Non HDL	9.8	ideally <4.0 mmol/l
LDL unable to be measured accurately because of high TG		

* ideally <2.5mmol/l refers to the general, healthy population. Importantly, lower targets may be indicated based on an individual patient's clinical situation.

For both sisters, the Australian Cardiovascular Disease Risk Calculator suggested a risk of an event of greater than 15 per cent in five years; their GPs recommended starting cholesterol treatment. After discussing the pros and cons of cardiac CT imaging to bring precision to their management decisions, both sisters proceeded with the testing. Their results follow.

CASE STUDY

Tracey

This is a zero calcium score and suggests a **low risk** of a coronary event in the next five to 10 years. This allowed for a conversation about cholesterol-lowering therapy that did not need to be at a high intensity, and a plan to rescan in five years.

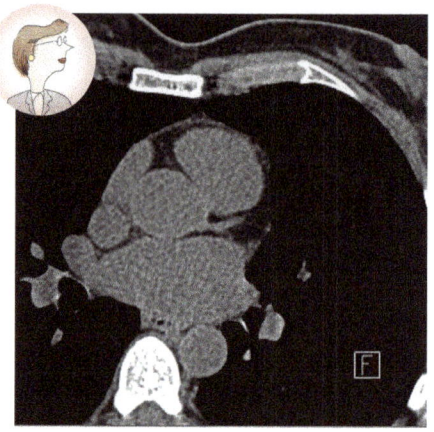

Tracy's scan for coronary artery calcium score

Beck

For Beck, the calcium score was over 1000. This score was very high and, in fact, the highest I have seen in a woman of this age. Compared with 100 women of the same age taken randomly from the population, she would be at least in the highest five (above the 95th percentile), perhaps even the most elevated. Beck's scans suggested **very high-risk** features and showed a significant plaque build-up in each of the three major arteries.

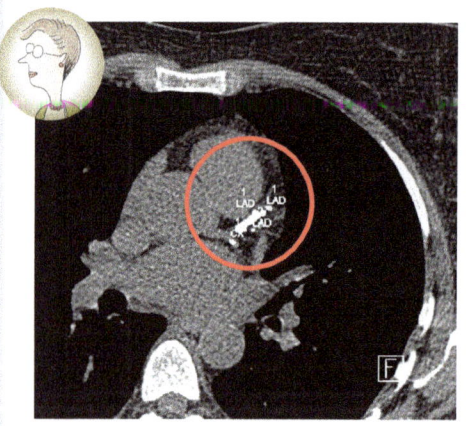
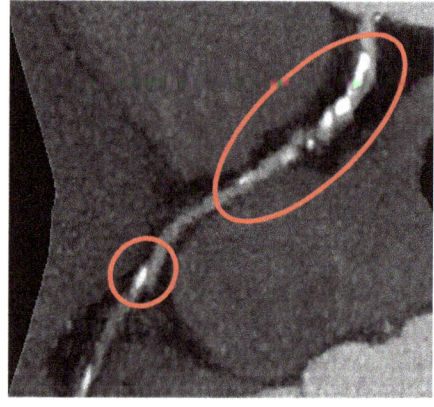

Beck's scan for coronary artery calcium score

Right coronary artery

These may be two sisters with the same family history and both with elevated cholesterol. However, the health of the arteries could not be more different. And no, I can't explain it. Nonetheless, the information was clear and allowed a management strategy based on **precisely** what was seen in the arteries, not a best guess based on a **population-based probability** of what might occur.

PATIENT PICTURES – TONY

CASE STUDY

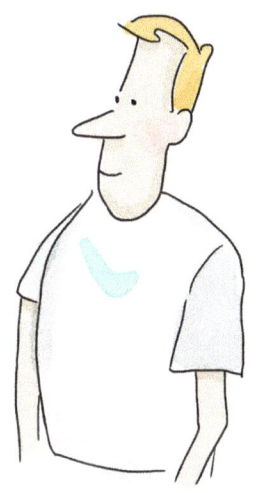

TONY was 63 years old when we met. He was proactive about his health and wanted to be as clear as possible about his cardiac risk. When I saw him, he was taking a cholesterol-lowering tablet, although it was a low dose and not aimed at the targets for a high-risk patient. He was not on aspirin. Interestingly, at his initiation, he had undergone two treadmill stress tests (through another centre) in the previous two years and had been reassured everything was fine. When he came to see me, he simply wanted as much information as possible to be clear he was addressing his cardiovascular risk appropriately.

This was his lipid profile:

Total Cholesterol (TC)	3.6	ideally < (less than) 5.0 mmol/l
Triglycerides (TG)	1.4	ideally <2.0 mmol/l
High Density Lipoprotein (HDL)	0.7	ideally > (greater than) 1.0 mmol/l
TC to HDL ratio	5.1	ideally <4.0 ratio
Non HDL	2.9	ideally <4.0 mmol/l
Low Density Lipoprotein (LDL)	2.2	ideally <2.5 mmol/l*

* ideally <2.5mmol/l refers to the general, healthy population. Importantly, lower targets may be indicated based on an individual patient's clinical situation.

These numbers look pretty good, so why worry. Still, we spoke at length, and Tony was eager to proceed to imaging his heart arteries for his peace of mind.

As you can see, (*next page*) he has a significant build-up. His calcium score was so high that it fell above the 90th percentile for his age group. The features were of **very high risk** of a coronary event.

With this information, we commenced aspirin, increased his lipid-lowering therapy, and improved his lipid profile in keeping with current guidelines. This information also provided valuable focus to maximise lifestyle changes.

CASE STUDY

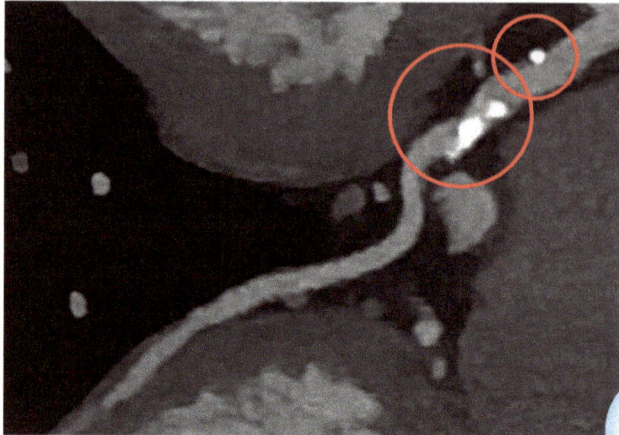

Tony's right coronary artery

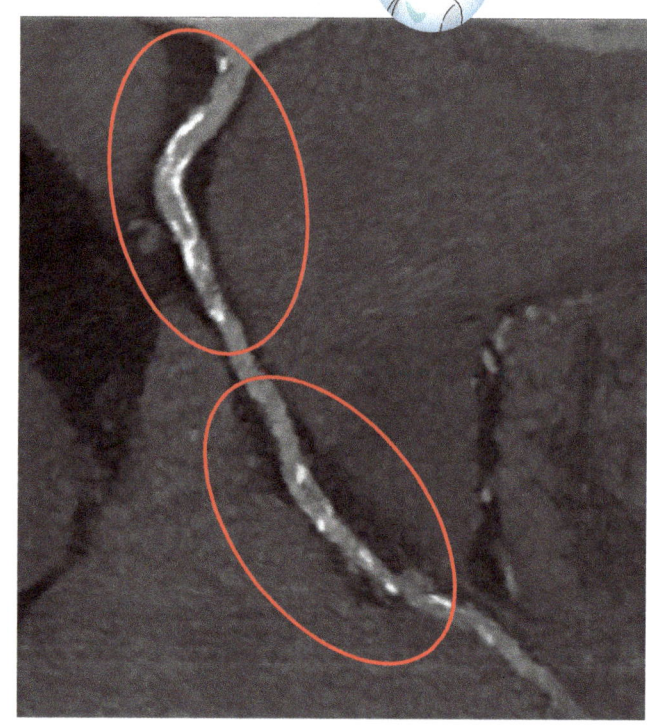

His circumflex artery

The other important factor is that Tony is now well educated. Should any symptom relating to his heart present, he knows to present for medical attention immediately. This education on its own could be life-saving.

Tony was delighted to have gone through the testing and to be better informed. There is no question that we have been able to improve his therapy concerning his actual risk based on the state of his arteries. He realised that the stress tests had told him that he was 'fit' but had not told him the 'fitness' of his arteries.

PATIENT PICTURES – PENNY (and her husband)   CASE STUDY

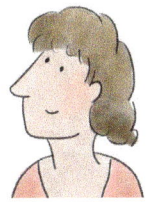

PENNY was 52 years old when she came to see me. She was generally well and on no medication. She was a non-smoker and didn't have elevated blood pressure. She was concerned, however, because she had a 'terrible' family history of premature coronary disease.

Her lipid profile was:

Total Cholesterol (TC)	6.1	ideally < (less than) 5.0 mmol/l
Triglycerides (TG)	0.6	ideally <2.0 mmol/l
High Density Lipoprotein (HDL)	2.1	ideally > (greater than) 1.0 mmol/l
TC to HDL ratio	2.1	ideally <4.0 ratio
Non HDL	4.0	ideally <4.0 mmol/l
Low Density Lipoprotein (LDL)	3.7	ideally <2.5 mmol/l*

* ideally <2.5mmol/l refers to the general, healthy population. Importantly, lower targets may be indicated based on an individual patient's clinical situation.

Putting these results into the Australian Cardiovascular Disease Risk Calculator gave Penny a risk estimated at one per cent in five years – a 'green light'.

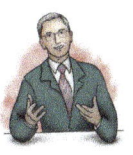

The important thing to remember here is that a risk calculator doesn't predict the risk for an individual patient. It provides the rate events occur in a group of 100 individuals with the same characteristics. This does not tell us who of the 100 will have the event.

Penny was well-informed when she came to see me. She had already had a significant discussion with her general practitioner and had looked at my website to obtain information about scanning the heart.

Her husband, who came with her, also decided to have his heart scanned. He was about the same age, with a similar lipid profile, had borderline high blood pressure and had a bit of weight on his tummy. He was the one who looked as if he might have the unhealthy arteries.

CASE STUDY

These were Penny's calcium score image and results:

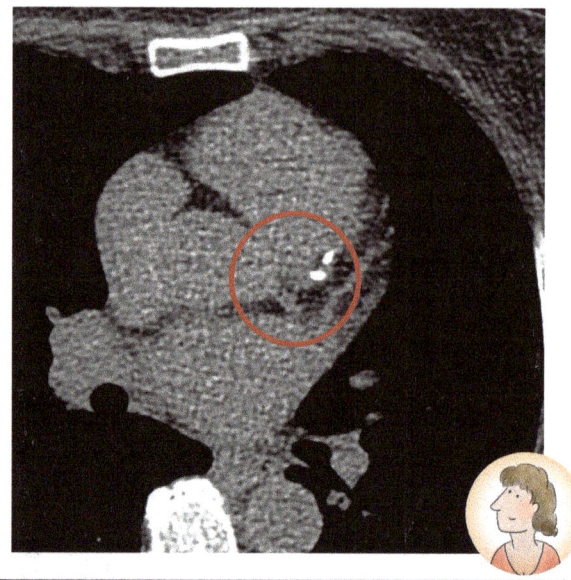

Penny's coronary artery calcium score image (right) and her results (below).

	LAD	LCX	RCA	Total Coronaries
Score	71.45	30.64	141.35	243.44
#POI's	2	2	14	18
AreaSq (sq.mm.)	17.86	12.77	46.22	76.85

Scoring Results : Agatston Score Protocol

The score of 243 is high for a young woman. For her age, the 90th percentile is 65! This result is three to four times higher, suggesting that Penny was probably the one out of the 100, the one per cent predicted to have an event in the next five years based on risk calculation. Not a 'green light' reassurance!

Although the result brought her to tears when she first heard this news, as the significance of having this knowledge sank in, she calmed down. There was no narrowing in the arteries, and there had been no damage to the heart. And, we had found what we had been looking for – to see if she had the same issues as others in her family. But, fortunately, although she did, **we had found the brake cylinder that was about to fail before the accident!**

We were able to institute appropriate therapy. For Penny, we were ahead of the game. There is little doubt Penny found this process confronting but invaluable and – I suggest – potentially lifesaving.

To complete the story, her husband had a zero calcium score!

coronary artery calcium score

So, what is this 'score' that is so significant in these case studies?

It has been noted earlier in the book that calcium – along with LDL cholesterol, scavenger cells and scar tissue – are the components of the atherosclerotic plaque that builds up in the coronary arteries leading to coronary artery disease (CAD), the forerunner to a heart attack.

Calcium has been observed in the arteries of living subjects for more than 80 years. While it is **not the problem**, it has become – through a test called a coronary artery calcium score, or CAC – the **standard marker** for indicating plaque build-up within the coronary arteries (atherosclerosis).

Calcium scoring provides a sensitive indicator to the presence of atheroma (the fatty deposits of plaque) within a person's arteries. It is an absolute number and there is a significant body of research that supports the premise that the greater the absolute coronary artery calcium score, then the greater the risk of an event that an individual carries.

I (WB) use the term coronary atheroma burden to describe finding plaque in the arteries of a patient who is otherwise well. It is a description for the extent of plaque formation within the coronary arteries as demonstrated on imaging before the development of disease. (In other words, a primary prevention setting.)

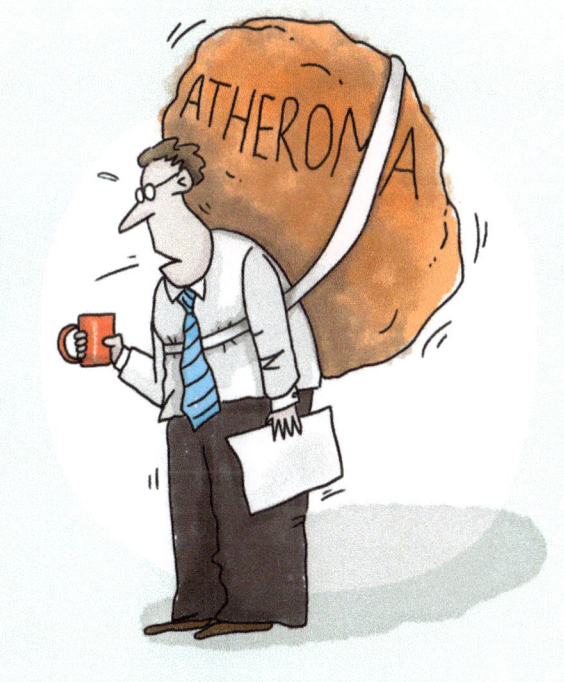

calcium

Calcium is not the problem. Calcium is inert in arteries, so it can stay there. However, it is an indicator of a potential risk. The problem is the plaque build-up of which calcium is a component.

Over many years, work in demonstrating an association between the amount of calcium present in an individual's arteries and the risk of progressing to a major adverse coronary event means that calcium scoring has become a prominent and sensible marker in risk assessment – a very powerful negative predictive test (meaning the condition is not present).

Neither a normal stress test (running on a treadmill), nor a normal invasive coronary angiogram (when the contrast or die is injected directly down the arteries) can provide the same assurance, while 'low cholesterol' 'regular exercise', 'good diet', 'watching my weight' and 'a healthy lifestyle' cannot come anywhere near to being as useful in predicting a low risk of an event as does a zero coronary artery calcium score.

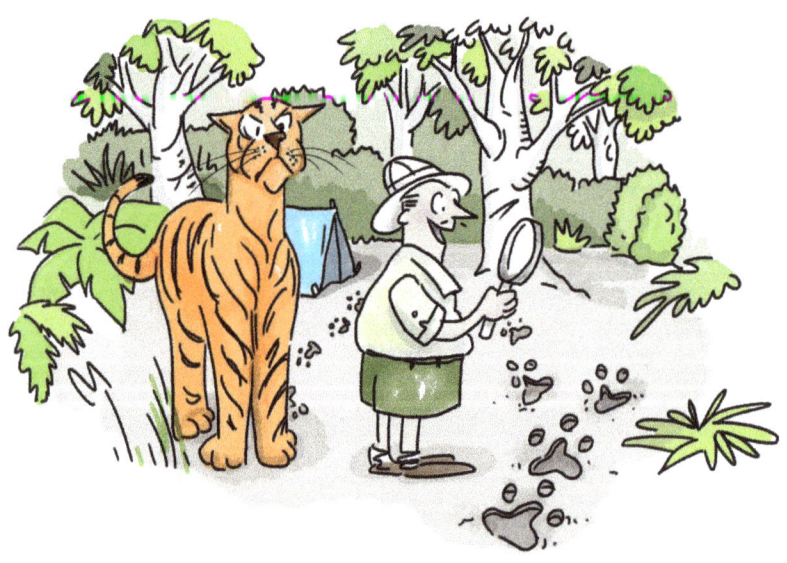

Calcium is simply the surrogate marker we use to give an indication of the process we are concerned about – the build-up of plaque within the coronary arteries. I (WB) use the example that if, on pitching a tent in the jungle, we saw lots of tiger footprints, it would mean that tigers are around, and it might not be a great place to pitch the tent. Not seeing tiger footprints doesn't mean there are not tigers in the area, but it certainly makes it a better place to pitch a tent! calcium is the tiger's footprint; atheroma is the tiger!

changing technology

In the 1980s, a new technology called **electron beam computed tomography** (EBCT) ignited renewed interest in evaluating the health of an individual's arteries. This so-called computed tomography (CT) has moved on a long way. Since about 2006, a new generation of CT machines has become available, gantry CT machines, and they continue to evolve.

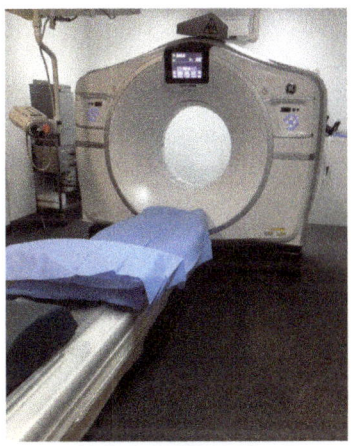

Today's CT scanners *(pictured right)* image the heart using a gantry system (a large ring) that spins x-ray heads and detectors around the patient at high-speed. Each rotation of image acquisition can obtain from four centimetres to the full vertical distance of the heart. The speed of rotation is very fast – and continues to increase with improvements in technology. Because the heart is constantly moving, the faster the image can be acquired, the less blur and the better quality of the image. These new machines, with more detectors and faster rotation times, are being used with advanced technologies that reduce the radiation doses to below ordinary yearly background radiation.

A CT scanner is used to measure the amount of calcium (calcified plaque) in the coronary arteries. A zero score indicates there is none.

what happens next?

The coronary artery calcium score (CAC) can be used in its own right, or as a gatekeeper to CT coronary angiography.

As we have seen, a zero score indicates that there is no calcium present in the arteries. Any score above zero is considered in relation to the person's age and sex.

If an abnormality is detected, then my general practice (WB) is to progress to CT coronary angiography (CTCA) to obtain as much information as possible about the health of the patient's coronary arteries and to consider plaque-specific factors. A CTCA, which involves injecting contrast into a vein in the arm, will outline the details of the arteries so that the structure and characteristics of individual plaque can be more thoroughly assessed.

The most significant feature now becomes the amount of cholesterol in the plaque.

cholesterol-dominant plaque

Cholesterol-dominant plaque, or **non-calcific** plaque, or **low attenuation plaque** (LAP), is the description of the build-up of lipid, or fat, within the plaque. The extent to which this occurs can have a significant bearing on the stability of the plaque. Our understanding around plaque rupture indicates that increasing lipid content is associated with less stability, and so a greater likelihood of rupture. Observational study shows that once a LAP is greater than eight millimetres in length and two millimetres in diameter (a LAP volume greater than 20mm³), it carries a significant and increased risk of event over the next few years.

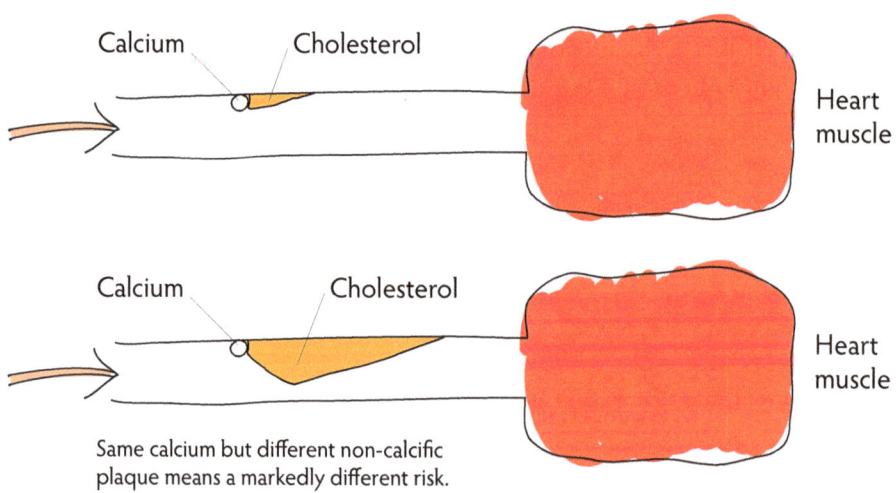

These diagrams show two similar spots of calcium in an artery, but they point to very different risk profiles due to the amount of associated cholesterol-laden plaque. The same calcium but different non-calcific plaque means a markedly different risk.

This is very important as it is possible to find significant LAP in the setting of a low CAC, and relatively low calcium score percentile. In this situation, the risk associated with the individual plaque becomes dominant in the future likelihood of the development of a major adverse coronary event for the individual patient.

The significance of this is that, although CAC is well validated for use in risk prediction, it can dramatically underestimate risk in patients who display non-calcific plaque depositions in excess of calcium deposition. This reiterates my point (WB) that the most comprehensive assessment of the health of the arteries, if calcium is demonstrated, is the combination of both CAC and CTCA, a complete 'cardiac scan'.

other factors

There are three other factors that come into play when considering plaque and risk:

- **remodelling** – the process in which the vessel changes shape, enlarging to accommodate the build-up of plaque within the artery wall;
- **stenosis** – narrowing of the artery;
- the **location** of the plaque within the coronary tree.

I (WB) discuss these features in more detail in my book, *Have You Planned Your Heart Attack?*
https://haveyouplannedyourheartattack.com.au/s/7ukaj

A CLOSER LOOK

stress testing

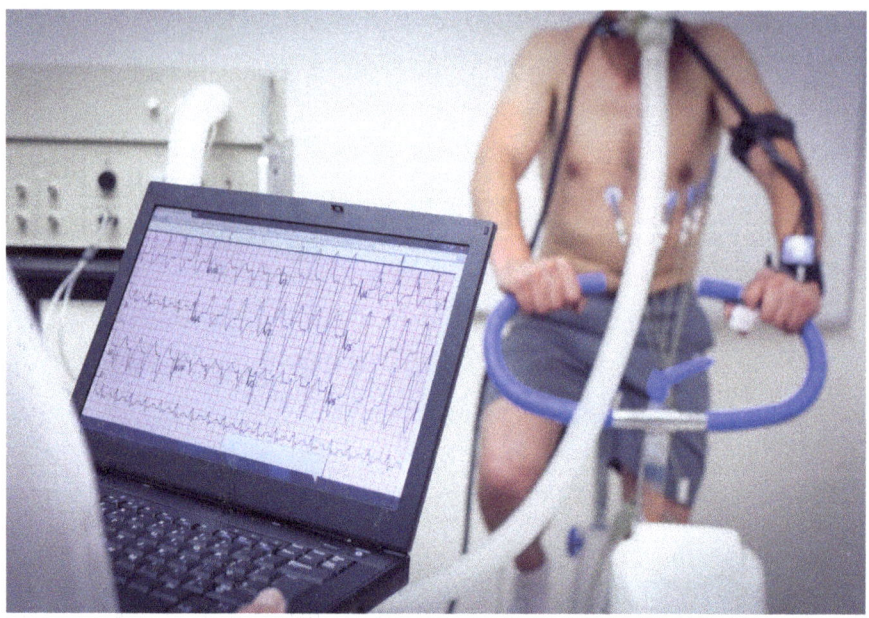

Stress testing is not considered standard practice for screening populations. It is acceptable to check your blood pressure, cholesterol, and other risk factors, but there is no standard recommendation for the general population to undergo stress testing. Occasionally, some patients come for stress testing in the context of risk stratification. I (WB) believe this provides some reassurance, but it is not necessarily good medicine.

It is interesting to note, however, that there are circumstances where stress testing is regularly undertaken: insurance companies still request stress testing, as does Motorsport Australia, that nation's governing body for motor racing, and the scientific Australian Antarctic Division. Some offshore workers need to fulfil occupational health and safety criteria, which include stress testing, and, most interestingly of all, the Civil Aviation Authority in Australia, still relies on stress testing for evaluating risk of commercial and private airline pilots, although CAC is starting to be used in routine CV risk screening for pilots.

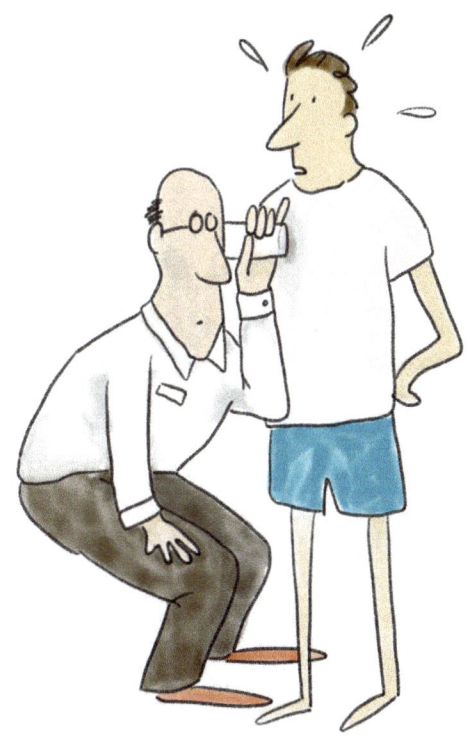

There are various stress testing modalities such as simple exercise stress tests (electrical trace of the heart activity – ECG), stress echocardiograms (in which we can see the heart – ECG + ultrasound of heart function), as well as pharmacological stress tests (using drugs to mimic exercise) for people who cannot walk.

Stress testing will only pick up evidence of narrowed coronary arteries – by which time it is **very late** in the process. And then, based on its **sensitivity** (the percentage of affected subjects detected by the test), it only picks up the problem at a rate of **75-80 per cent**, meaning that it will miss one-in-five to one-in-six occurrences. Cardiac CT sensitivity, however, is **over 98 per cent**. Such a high percentage means it might miss only one in 50, making it a very sensitive test. Sensitive and specific.

As well as not being particularly accurate, the stress test makes no appraisal of non-flow-limiting coronary atheroma burden, which has been demonstrated to be the culprit for coronary occlusion (by rupture of the plaque, leading to blockage from the formation of a clot in the artery) in more than 40 per cent of cases.

This means, if stress testing detects 75 per cent of narrowed arteries accurately and zero per cent of non-narrowed arteries, and if 60 per cent of heart attacks occur on narrowed arteries, stress testing is detecting 75 per cent of 60 per cent of the plaque that will lead to a problem, giving a pickup rate of less than 45 per cent (60 per cent x 75 per cent). A toss of the coin provides a better detection rate (50 per cent), by chance, alone!

PATIENT PICTURES – BILL A CLOSER LOOK

Bill, aged 48, requested cardiac CT imaging in the context of a family history of premature coronary artery disease.

Scanning demonstrated a high CAC, in fact, above the 90th percentile for age and sex. We undertook stress testing to assess for possible flow limitation. This did not suggest tightly narrowed arteries.

After also undergoing screening bloods for high-risk factors, Bill started taking aspirin, a statin, an ACE inhibitor, vitamin D and fish oil. Regular exercise and reduced carbohydrate eating were also part of the regime.

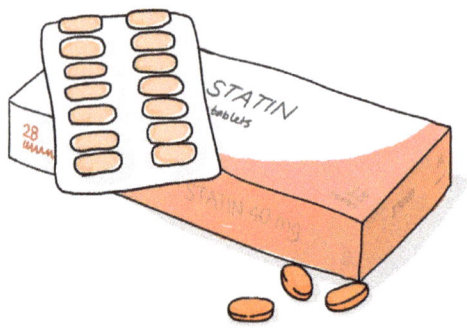

Unfortunately, Bill did not tolerate the statin well. Still, we persisted with as much statin as he could tolerate, a very low dose, every second or third day.

In the context of not being able to treat as we had hoped nor achieve the desired lower lipid levels, we discussed undertaking serial surveillance stress testing as a potential indicator of progression that could lead to narrowing of the arteries.

The electrocardiogram (ECG) demonstrated some change suggestive of narrowed arteries. Still, there was no evidence of regional wall motion abnormality (the heart muscle worked well, suggesting good blood supply to most of the heart). We repeated the test about a year later with similar results, with no lessening in exercise capacity.

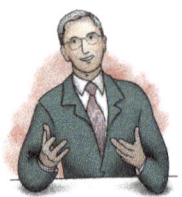

Please note, this is different to using stress testing to define risk. Here we already knew the risk from the cardiac scan and used the stress testing to assess if any of the arteries were narrowing.

Another year on, we repeated the stress echocardiogram. On this occasion, it clearly demonstrated the presence of regional wall motion abnormality (the muscle 'cramps' from lack of blood, becomes stiff, and fails to pump properly), affecting the posterior wall, most likely affected by the circumflex artery. Bill had some mild shortness of breath but, because of his excellent exercise capacity, performed very well on the test. Nonetheless, the extent of affected muscle was such that I believed we should progress to invasive coronary angiography to consider potential revascularisation.

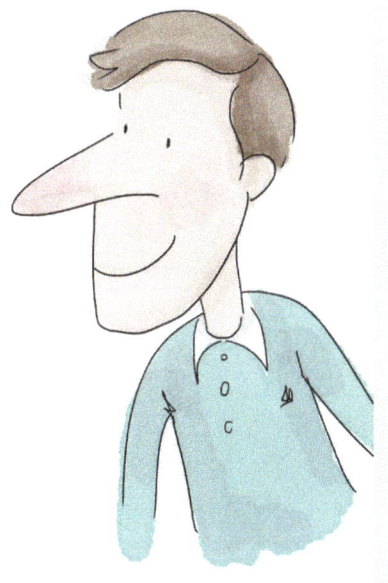

Within the week, Bill had undergone invasive coronary angiography, and had a stent inserted in the proximal circumflex artery, which resulted in fully re-established blood flow to that area of the heart. He was back at work several days later. There was no damage to his heart. He resumed full work and exercise capacity and is again wrestling with trying to take statins. We plan to continue with follow-up stress testing.

As an aside, we scanned other members of his family, and we are appropriately risk-managing them, although their risks were not as high as Bill's.

Bill represents, I believe, one of the potential 15 out of the 100 who would otherwise have been 'in the crowd' of **intermediate risk** had we not identified him.

His alternative scenario may have been sudden cardiac death or to have presented with a heart attack. The latter could have led to a terrifying ride in the back of an ambulance, Accident and Emergency time, an out-of-hours call to open the invasive angiography unit, followed by a scary ICU stay. In addition, damage to his myocardium might have prevented him from returning to the exercise he enjoys, limited his lifestyle, kept him from work, and, if the damage were significant, may have required the implantation of a defibrillating device. The costs – emotional, financial and time – could have been enormous.

IMPORTANT POINTS

SHOULD WE GUESS OR TAKE A LOOK?

- A risk calculator gives the rate of an event in a population with the same traditional risk factors, not the risk for the individual.
- Imaging the arteries brings precision to an individual assessment.
- See below for further important action information.

For a **FREE HEART HEALTH CHECK** and to **PURCHASE** a **SCAN** if appropriate, please visit: https://drwarrickbishop.com/s/vhc

 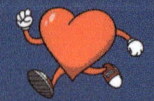

Further information is available in Dr Bishop's book – *Have You Planned Your Heart Attack?*
https://drwarrickbishop.com/s/books

 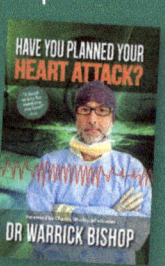

High cholesterol levels require treatment.

chapter 12
DEALING WITH CHOLESTEROL

The body **needs** cholesterol as it is a building block of the walls of all our cells. Cholesterol is also important in producing hormones, vitamin D and bile. Manufactured, naturally, in the liver, it is water-insoluble and floats around the body so that if left to its own devices, it would float to the 'surface' like cream in a bottle of unhomogenised milk. **Lipoproteins** (particles comprised of protein and fat) carry cholesterol from the liver through the blood to the tissues and back from the tissues to the liver. While most cholesterol is formed **naturally** within the body, it is also in the **foods** we eat. Although cholesterol is essential for building healthy cells, the risk of developing heart disease – blocked blood vessels, heart attack, stroke – rises and falls with the rise and fall of cholesterol levels in the blood. One in 250-300 people are born with a condition called **familial hypercholesterolemia.** These people have very high blood cholesterol levels from birth and often will develop heart disease in their 40s or 50s.

the good, the bad, the ugly, and the very ugly

Four factors are essential concerning the body's cholesterol levels:
- low-density lipoprotein (LDL) – 'bad'
  - most of the body's cholesterol is LDL, the so-called 'bad' cholesterol. It can stick to the walls of arteries and help cause the fatty build-up, plaque. Too much plaque leads to blockages of the arteries, preventing enough blood from flowing to the heart – the cause of a heart attack.
- high-density lipoprotein (HDL) – 'good'
  - as HDL cholesterol carries LDL cholesterol away from the arteries and back to the liver to be broken down and passed from the body as waste, it is often called 'good' cholesterol.

normal

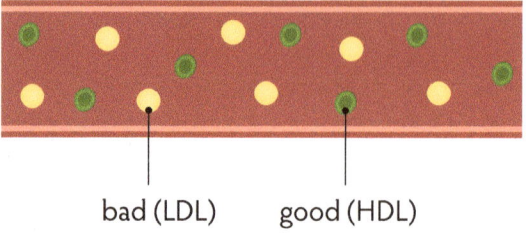

bad (LDL)   good (HDL)

atherosclerosis

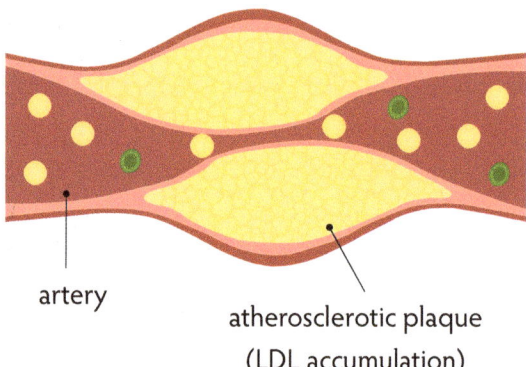

artery   atherosclerotic plaque
(LDL accumulation)

- triglycerides – 'ugly'
  - triglycerides are the most common fat in the body. Along with increased LDL cholesterol or decreased HDL cholesterol, they can increase the chances of developing fatty build-ups in the arteries, plaque, leading to a higher risk of heart attack or stroke.
- lipoprotein (a) – 'very ugly'
  - lipoprotein (a), Lp(a), is a lipoprotein that looks and behaves like LDL with another protein called apo (a) attached to it. This additional protein makes Lp(a) more problematic than LDL, as it increases the chance of blood clots, is more likely to deposit in the arteries, can trigger inflammation, and can even accelerate wear and tear of the aortic valve. It is a robust risk factor and is genetically determined. Twenty per cent of the population has high Lp(a) levels.

While cholesterol levels are mainly related to genetic factors, they are also clearly associated with lifestyle factors, particularly consumption of saturated fat, sugar and alcohol, lack of exercise, being overweight, smoking and having high blood pressure. *(continued page 160)*

PATIENT PICTURES – JOHN CASE STUDY

JOHN was a 35-year-old male with high cholesterol who had tried cholesterol-lowering tablets but had suffered aches and pains. He didn't want to be on medication unless it was clearly indicated.

At our first meeting, he was fit, well, and not on any regular medication. His family had no history of premature coronary artery disease, although his parents had elevated cholesterol.

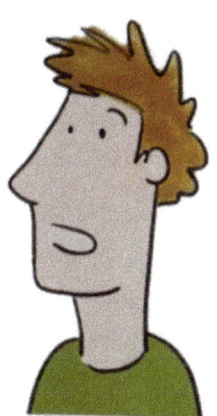

His lipid profile was:

Total Cholesterol (TC)	11.0	ideally < (less than) 5.0 mmol/l
Triglycerides (TG)	1.9	ideally <2.0 mmol/l
High Density Lipoprotein (HDL)	1.0	ideally > (greater than) 1.0 mmol/l
TC to HDL ratio	11.0	ideally <4.0 ratio
Non HDL	10.0	ideally <4.0 mmol/l
Low Density Lipoprotein (LDL)	9.1	ideally <2.5 mmol/l*

* ideally <2.5mmol/l refers to the general, healthy population. Importantly, lower targets may be indicated based on an individual patient's clinical situation.

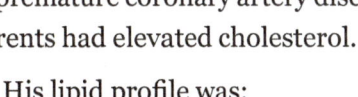

These levels of cholesterol are high and concerning. The Australian Absolute Cardiovascular Disease Risk Calculator determined John's risk at greater than a 15 per cent chance of an event in the next five years or over 30 per cent in 10 years. These figures suggest a **very high risk**.

We spoke at some length about the role of scanning his heart to provide more information about the state of his arteries to determine in more detail what his risk might be. I explained that he was younger than usual for such scanning. I also explained the danger of x-ray exposure (about the same or less than a mammogram).

John was keen to undergo scanning to be as well-informed as possible and make the best decisions for his care. He was married with three children and didn't want to leave his heart health to chance.

CASE STUDY

The calcium score was three. In absolute terms, this score is not high, yet over the 75th percentile for his age. In combination with his cholesterol levels, it was high enough to support lowering his cholesterol for a safer future.

This information was what John needed to know to be clear about his health management. I indicated that he would benefit from treatment. The pictures were explicit; gone were his doubts about the benefits of the medication.

He is now on aspirin and two cholesterol-lowering medications and has also embraced significant lifestyle changes. The result is a major turnaround in the management of his cardiovascular risk. He is happy with the outcome – of being informed and proactive.

PATIENT PICTURES – KAREN

KAREN was a 60-year-old woman who came to see me for cardiovascular risk stratification. She was generally fit and well, not on any regular medication, and there was no history of premature coronary artery disease in her family.

Her lipid profile was:

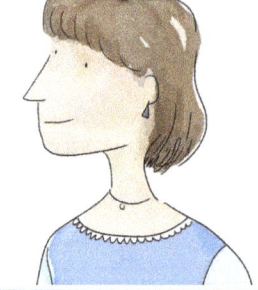

Total Cholesterol (TC)	9.1	ideally < (less than) 5.0 mmol/l
Triglycerides (TG)	2.0	ideally <2.0 mmol/l
High Density Lipoprotein (HDL)	2.1	ideally > (greater than) 1.0 mmol/l
TC to HDL ratio	4.3	ideally <4.0 ratio
Non HDL	7.0	ideally <4.0 mmol/l
Low Density Lipoprotein (LDL)	6.1	ideally <2.5 mmol/l*

*ideally <2.5mmol/l refers to the general, healthy population. Importantly, lower targets may be indicated based on an individual patient's clinical situation.

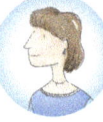

CASE STUDY

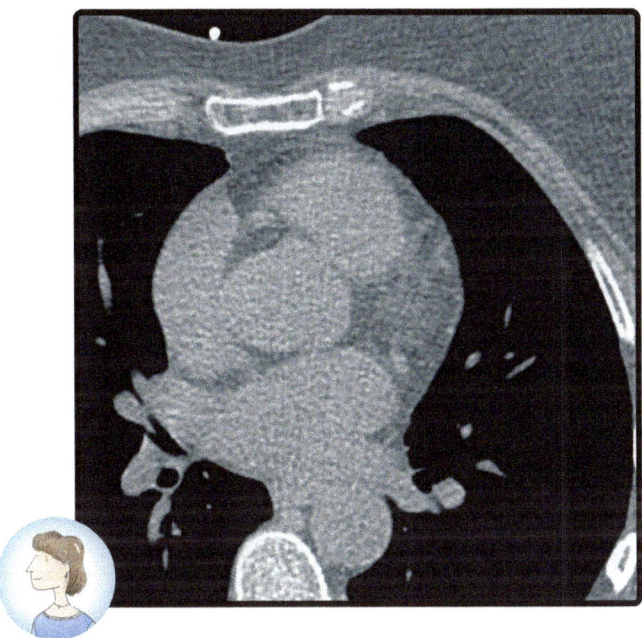

This is the scan result for Karen.

Her coronary artery calcium score was zero. There was no evidence of plaque build-up, despite her elevated cholesterol levels.

Karen experienced fantastic relief. Her doctor's desire to have her on a cholesterol-lowering tablet, notwithstanding the side effects she suffered, had stressed her – catching her between the fear of an event and the side effects of medication.

Based on the above scan, I reassured her that the available research suggested that a zero calcium score represented a **very low-risk** – a risk of an event of less than one per cent in five years (all things being equal). We discussed this at some length and agreed on a plan of management – low doses of cholesterol treatment, and ongoing surveillance.

A demonstrated low risk of an event informed the immediate medication decision.

A plan for ongoing surveillance supported this action.

Karen was happy with the outcome.

(from page 156)

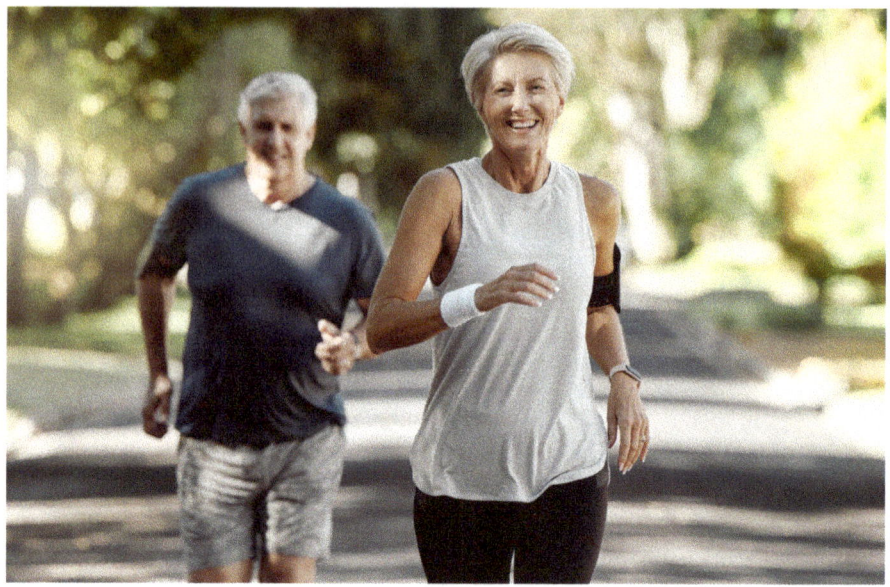

More than two in five (41.9 per cent) Australian adults live with high cholesterol, which peaks among those aged between 55 and 64.

The three ways of lowering cholesterol are

- diet and nutraceuticals
  - some foods are higher in cholesterol and saturated fats than others, or they may contain ingredients that can contribute to high cholesterol.
  - nutraceuticals (dietary supplements, functional food), such as plant sterols, fibre and soy, can lower cholesterol.
- physical activity
  - physical activity can help raise 'good' cholesterol levels (HDL) and lower triglycerides. Aerobic or cardio exercise and resistance training are beneficial for controlling cholesterol levels. *(see chapter 6)*
- medication
  - medication can help improve a cholesterol profile, thus reducing the risk of a heart attack. Follow your doctor's advice and take the medication as directed. **Do not stop** because you feel better. The medicine will continue to work in the background to keep your cholesterol under control.

medications

Commonly used medications to control cholesterol are:

- **statins** are a class of medications that helps lower cholesterol levels by inhibiting the enzyme HMG-CoA reductase, which is involved in cholesterol synthesis in the liver.
  - examples, atorvastatin, simvastatin, and rosuvastatin;
- **ezetimibe** works by reducing the absorption of cholesterol from the diet in the small intestine. It is often used in combination with statins for individuals who require further cholesterol reduction.
- **proprotein convertase subtilisin/kexin type 9** (PCSK9) **inhibitors** are a newer class of medications that help lower LDL cholesterol levels by blocking the protein, PCSK9. This protein regulates the number of LDL receptors on liver cells, and by inhibiting it, PCSK9 inhibitors increase the liver's ability to clear LDL cholesterol from the bloodstream. They are generally used in association with statins, although they can sometimes be a stand-alone drug therapy.

As high cholesterol does not have apparent symptoms, your doctor must check your levels **regularly** through blood testing.

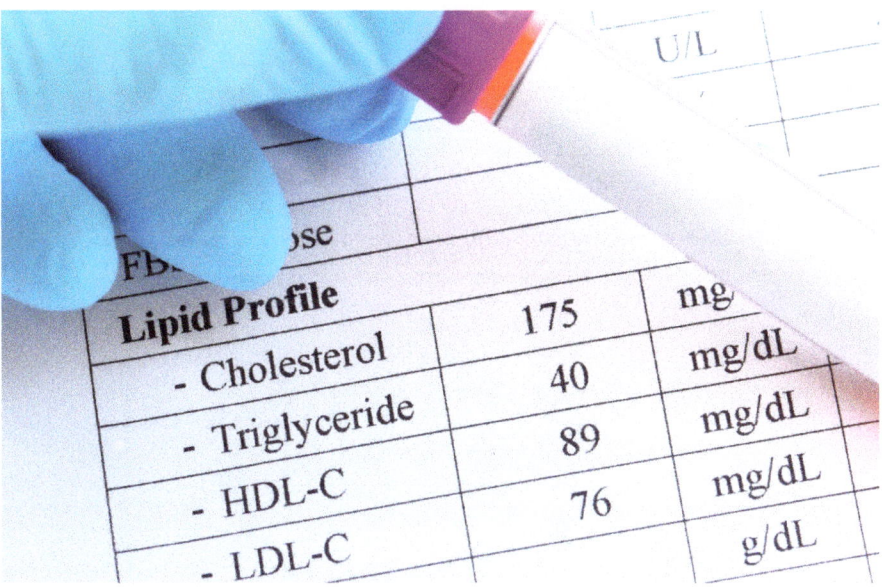

in Australia and the United Kingdom, the results of a lipid profile are usually reported in millimoles per litre (mmol/l), while in the USA, the units used are milligrams per deciliter (mg/dL)

IMPORTANT POINTS

DEALING WITH CHOLESTEROL

- Most cholesterol is produced naturally within the liver and is essential to body health.
- High cholesterol is an association of plaque, meaning that high cholesterol levels do not always denote that plaque is present in the arteries.
- Three ways of lowering cholesterol are:
  - diet and nutraceuticals,
  - physical activity, and
  - medication.
- As high cholesterol does not have any obvious symptoms, it is important that your levels are checked regularly.
- Imaging the arteries can offer valuable individualised information in relation to high cholesterol.
  (Please refer back to chapter 11.)

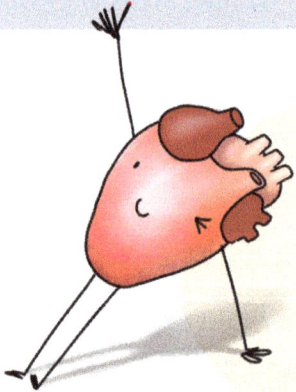

Change is possible, especially:

- ☒ with the help of education
- ☒ through seeking medical advice
- ☒ asking for the support and encouragement of others.

Aspirin is the world's most used drug.
Yet, its long-term use is not for everyone.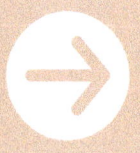

chapter 13
ASPIRIN – FRIEND OR FOE?

Aspirin, the household word for a drug known around the world, is the registered name for acetylsalicylic acid. This organic compound with the chemical formula $C_9H_8O_4$, was developed by the German pharmaceutical company Bayer in the late 1800s. The name 'aspirin' was registered in 1899. However, for the preceding two millennia, a group of chemicals, salicylates,[76] all found naturally in the leaves of the willow tree, provided a therapeutic benefit.

Since the refining of acetylsalicylic acid and the marketing of aspirin, its use has become widespread and currently is the most widely used medical preparation in the world. About 100 billion pills are produced each year.

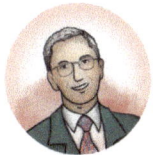

These are almost incomprehensible numbers but when you stop to think about what it can do, it starts to make some sense.

prostaglandins

Aspirin works by blocking an enzyme called **cyclooxygenase**, which then alters production of other compounds called **prostaglandins** that act as chemical messengers throughout the body. This alteration creates numerous impacts within the body.

- Prostaglandins within the brain influence the way fevers develop. If you are in bed with the flu and have a fever, taking a couple of aspirin (blocking cyclooxygenase) will lower the prostaglandins (responsible for the fever) and your temperature will go down.
- Prostaglandins have a role in appreciation of pain and the way pain receptors respond. So, if you have a headache (perhaps with your fever) then blocking your cyclooxygenase and altering your prostaglandin production will ease the pain.

- Prostaglandins also influence the way blood vessels respond to inflammation. If you have a sore arthritic knee from too much work in the garden, the associated swelling could be reduced by blocking the cyclooxygenase, reducing the prostaglandins involved in the inflammatory response.

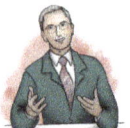

For pain, fever, and inflammation it is pretty handy to keep a box of aspirin in the cupboard to use on an as-needed basis. I am sure we have taken relief by manipulating our prostaglandins using a cyclooxygenase blocking agent – taking a couple of aspirin – and going to bed.

- Prostaglandins also help protect the lining of the stomach from acid. Using aspirin for any length of time may change the prostaglandins within the stomach, leading to less resistance to the formation of an ulcer.
    - Long-term use of aspirin may also cause bleeding within the gastrointestinal tract. A couple of tablets when we have a headache or a sore throat or even a fever with flu-like symptoms will not have detrimental effects on the gastric or upper gastrointestinal lining. Ongoing, continued impact on the prostaglandins could cause problems. However, there are some reasons that may outweigh the risk of side effects.

platelets

Aspirin helps reduce the stickiness of platelets. Platelets are the small particles in the blood needed for the formation of clots. These small particles are activated when there is any irregularity within the blood vessel. For example, in a cut, foreign material encounters the 'coagulant' proteins in the bloodstream that sets off a 'cascade' of activation in which the platelets clump with the coagulant proteins to form a clot. A ruptured plaque within an artery – the mechanism for a heart attack – exposes foreign material (proteins in the vessel wall) to the platelets and the coagulation proteins, activating them to combine, and a clot forms (*refer back to pages 48-49*).

studies

That reducing platelet stickiness reduces the risk of a heart attack has been demonstrated many times since 1988.

ISIS-2

Some 30 years ago, the ISIS-2 trial[77] showed that giving aspirin to patients very soon after a heart attack reduced the likelihood of that patient having a heart attack in the future compared to not giving aspirin.

That first trial demonstrating aspirin's benefit has been followed by many others, all of them in the setting of preventing **a second event** and all of them showing **benefit** in terms of reducing risk of subsequent heart attack. These trials involved **high-risk** patients.

Where controversy has simmered, subsequently, is whether giving aspirin to people **before** they have an event – that is in the **primary prevention** setting before they have declared themselves as very high risk – offers any benefit. Around 2018 several trials were released that tried to answer this question.

ASCEND

The ASCEND trial[78], published in *American Heart Journal*, studied patients who were diabetic but did not have any history of heart problems – a primary prevention population. Fifteen thousand patients were followed for more than seven years. Although there was a suggestion that the risk of having a heart attack was reduced in the aspirin group, this benefit was offset by an increased risk of bleeding from the upper part of the gut or into the brain, caused by being on the drug long-term. The ASCEND trial did **not** show benefit in giving aspirin to a group of diabetic patients who had not had previous heart problems.

ARRIVE

Released about the same time as the ASCEND trial results but in a different publication, *The Lancet,* a study called ARRIVE[79] showed that aspirin had **no** significant benefit in outcome when given to 13,000 patients randomised to aspirin or not. These people had moderate cardiovascular risk (between 10 and 20 per cent risk of an event in 10 years) but had not had a previous heart attack or stroke. These patients were followed for about six years during which time any benefits in reduction of stroke or heart attack were matched by complications of bleeding.

ASPREE

The most recent of these aspirin-in-primary-prevention trials was the ASPREE[80] trial. This enrolled nearly 20,000 people across the world in an attempt to evaluate whether aspirin, given to otherwise healthy older adults over 70 years of age, would improve function and reduce death. After following these participants for about six years, there was no suggestion that giving aspirin to this healthy group of older citizens made any difference. There was even a small suggestion that it could worsen outcomes. It is worth noting that these healthy older adults had become healthy older adults because they hadn't had coronary artery or cardiovascular disease until that point and, so, to some degree, had been potentially self-selected as a relatively low risk group to benefit from aspirin in the context of reducing cardiovascular risk.

using aspirin

So where does all this information leave us now?

Aspirin should **not** be used to try and reduce risk of heart attack and stroke for everyone. **It does not have a clear-cut indication in normal primary preventative situations of low or moderate/intermediate risk patients.** Some data suggest that patients with elevated blood pressure **may** benefit from being on aspirin, probably because elevated blood pressure can push people into a higher risk category.

I (WB) try to be more precise about evaluating an individual's risk in a primary preventative setting by undertaking imaging of the coronary arteries *(as described in chapter 11)*. As none of the primary prevention studies above incorporated imaging as a selector for aspirin therapy or not, any question about the use of imaging and aspirin in primary prevention remains unanswered. My feeling, however, is that if, through imaging, we find people with high or very high-risk features then, understanding the pros and cons of aspirin and based on the individual's situation, it may be a reasonable consideration. This is something that needs to be pondered on a patient-by-patient basis with all the information available and with a clear conversation between doctor and patient striving for the best management strategy for that individual[81].

When it comes to **secondary** prevention, that is people who have had a heart attack or stroke, there remains **no question that aspirin is beneficial.**

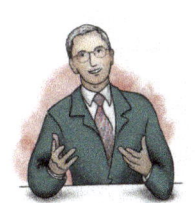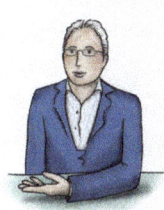

If you have had a problem with your heart arteries, neck arteries or the arteries in the legs (peripheral vascular disease, PVD), and you have been put on aspirin by your doctor, that aspirin is doing a good job for you. Please do not stop your therapy based on how the ASCEND, ARRIVE and ASPREE trials have been presented by some media. Please check with your medical practitioner or specialist about how it relates to you.

other medications

After experiencing a heart attack, you will be prescribed a cocktail of medications to help manage your condition and reduce the risk of future cardiovascular events.

While your specific medications will depend on your circumstances and your medical history, some common post heart attack medications include:

- **antiplatelet drugs** are prescribed to prevent blood clots from forming, thus reducing the risk of another heart attack or stroke.
    - examples, aspirin, clopidogrel;
- **beta-blockers** to help lower blood pressure and reduce the workload on the heart, making it easier for the heart to pump blood effectively. They also reduce the risk of arrhythmia in the first year after a heart attack thus reducing the risk of SCD (examples, *see page 124*);
- **angiotensin-converting enzyme inhibitors** (ACE inhibitors) relax blood vessels and decrease blood pressure, and so reduce the strain on the heart (examples, *see page 124*);
- **statins** lower cholesterol levels and reduce the risk of plaque build-up in arteries, which can lead to atherosclerosis and a heart attack.
    - examples, atorvastatin, simvastatin, rosuvastatin;
- **nitroglycerin** is often used to relieve chest pain (angina) and improve blood flow to the heart;
- **angiotensin II receptor blockers** (ARBs) also help relax the blood vessels and lower blood pressure (examples, *see page 124)*;
- **diuretics** help reduce fluid build-up and lower blood pressure by increasing urine production (examples, *see page 124*);
- **anticoagulants** help prevent blood clots and reduce the risk of stroke especially in patients with certain heart conditions such as atrial fibrillation.
    - examples, warfarin or the newer oral anticoagulants including apixaban, dabigatran and rivaroxaban;
- **calcium channel blockers** help relax and widen blood vessels, thus reducing blood pressure and improving blood flow (examples, *see page 124*).

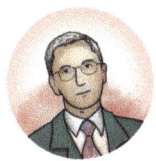 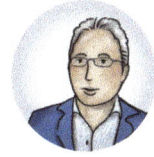

Every treatment needs to be considered for the individual patient based on the benefit of that therapy weighed clearly against the inherent risks.

Please work with your doctor for your own best outcomes. Always follow your doctor's advice and take medications as prescribed to effectively manage your heart health and reduce the risk of future heart events.

IMPORTANT POINTS

ASPIRIN – FRIEND OR FOE?

- Aspirin is the most widely used medical preparation in the world.
- Aspirin can be useful for reducing fever and pain.
- Long-term use of aspirin carries the risk of bleeding. However, this can be offset in certain circumstances by its benefit in reducing the risk of heart attack or stroke.
- All patients with CVD / stroke and peripheral vascular disease should be on aspirin (or an aspirin-like agent) unless there is a good reason not to be.
- Ongoing use of aspirin needs medical supervision and should not be self-prescribed.
- Aspirin is one of many drugs that will be prescribed to manage your condition and reduce the risk of future cardiovascular events.

76	*Salicylates are natural chemicals made by fruits and vegetables and help protect plants against disease and insects.*
77	*Randomised trial of intravenous streptokinase, oral aspirin, both, or neither among 17,187 cases of suspected acute myocardial infarction: ISIS – 2 Published: August 13, 1988. The Lancet. (source: https://www.thelancet.com/journals/lancet/article/PIIS0140-6736(88)92833-4/fulltext)*
78	*ASCEND: A Study of Cardiovascular Events iN Diabetes: Characteristics of a randomised trial of aspirin and of omega-three fatty acid supplementation in 15,480 people with diabetes. Am Heart J 2018 Apr;198:135-144.* *doi: 10.1016/j.ahj.2017.12.006. 10.1016/j.ahj.2017.12.006. Epub 2017 Dec 24.* *(source: https://pubmed.ncbi.nlm.nih.gov/29653635/)*
79	*Use of aspirin to reduce risk of initial vascular event in patients at moderate risk of cardiovascular disease (ARRIVE): a randomised, double blind, placebo-controlled trial. Published: August 26, 2018. (source: https://www.thelancet.com/article/S0140-6736(18)31924-X/fulltext)*
80	*please refer to: Effect of Aspirin on All-Cause Mortality in the Healthy Elderly, N Engl J Med 2018; 379:1519-1528 DOI: 10.1056/NEJMoa1803955 (https://www.nejm.org/doi/full/10.1056/nejmoa1803955)*
81	*Dr Bishop's book, Have You Planned Your Heart Attack? (Know Your Real Risk of Heart Attack, in the USA) is about the power of imaging in preventative cardiology.*

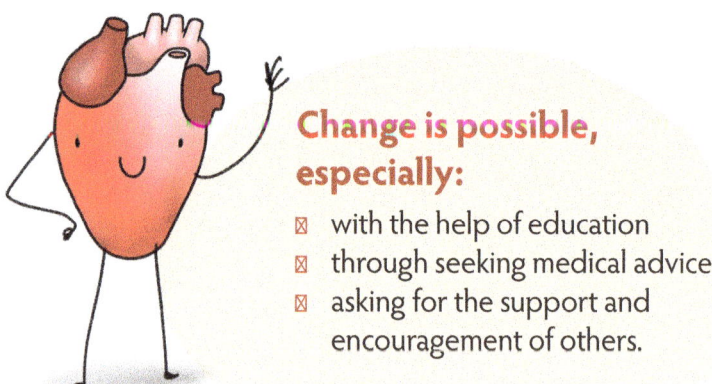

Change is possible, especially:

- with the help of education
- through seeking medical advice
- asking for the support and encouragement of others.

Pursuing cardiac health should not be a loan or lonely pursuit.

chapter 14
TEAMWORK

Teamwork may be the shortest chapter in the book, but it is one of the most important – if you want to successfully lower your risk of having a heart attack or other coronary event or disease.

In a previous book, *Cardiac Rehabilitation Explained* (2023), we (WB and Dr Alistair Begg) emphasised the importance of having people – family, friends and health professionals – support a person in rehabilitation after an event or illness. Essentially, rehabilitation aims at preventing a second occurrence and having the patient live as healthy and active a life for as long as possible. Although this book is mainly about preventing the **first** occurrence, particularly a heart attack, much of the mindset is similar.

Good habits – and, if necessary, **change** – are **essential.**

As we have seen throughout this book, most risk factors involve lifestyle choices. An honest answer to these questions – *Do I need to change*, and, *Am I prepared to change?* – is the beginning of taking care of yourself, of effective long-term improved health. The way forward is a forked road:

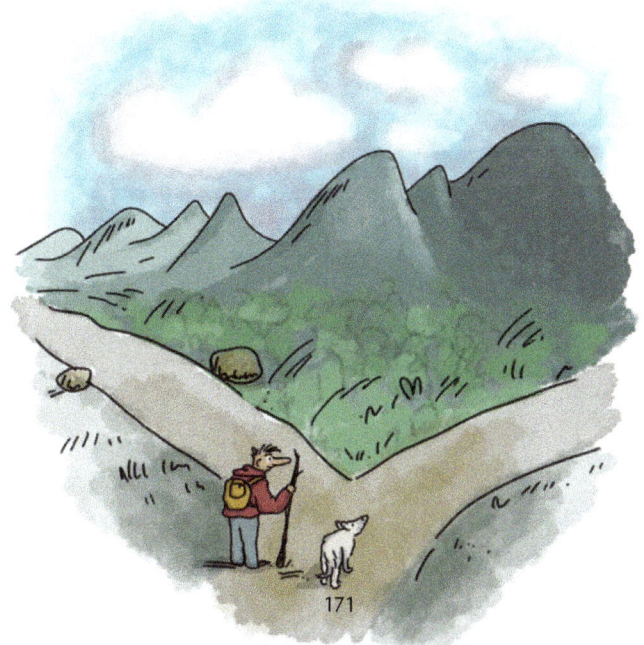

- do you live with your high-risk factors, which are likely to cause a heart attack or worsen cardiac disease, or
- do you embrace new life choices as the beginning of new habits for a better quality of life and a healthier lifestyle?

Change is never comfortable, straightforward, or easy. For many of us, instant gratification through food, drink, and a bit longer on the couch is much easier than worrying about something we can't feel or see. Not today, anyway.

While there is no question that **prevention is better than cure** when it comes to a heart attack, unfortunately for many, the 'best will in the world' needs some help. The **good news** is that there is plenty of help available.

Your team members could include:

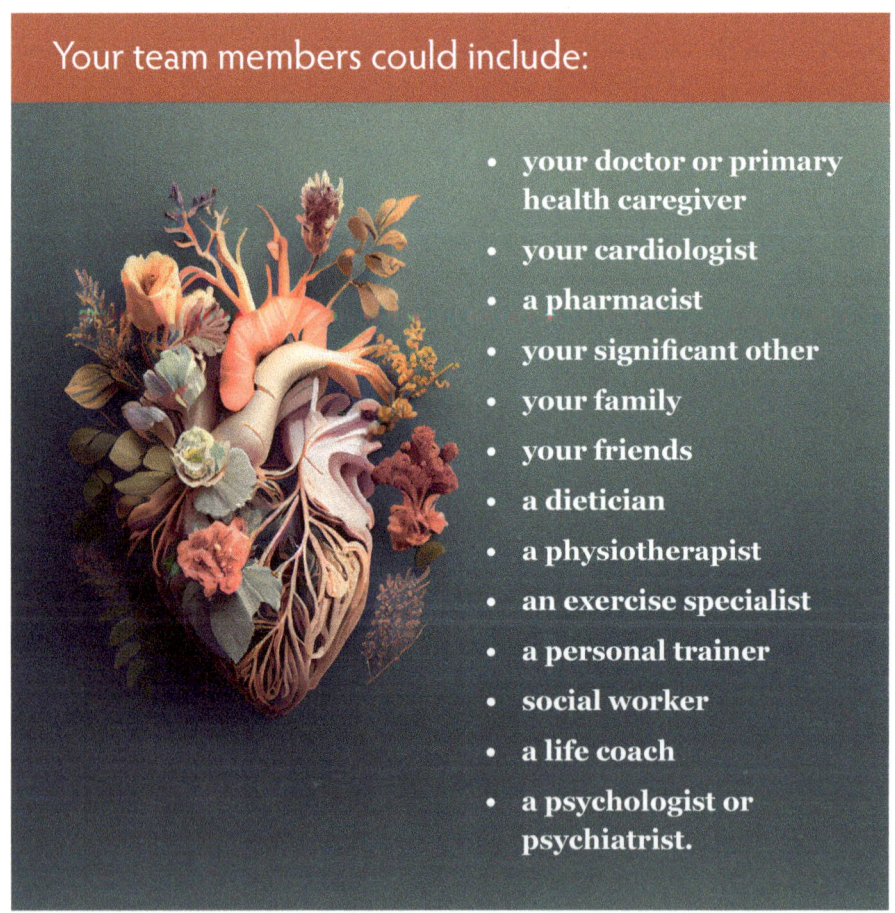

- **your doctor or primary health caregiver**
- **your cardiologist**
- **a pharmacist**
- **your significant other**
- **your family**
- **your friends**
- **a dietician**
- **a physiotherapist**
- **an exercise specialist**
- **a personal trainer**
- **social worker**
- **a life coach**
- **a psychologist or psychiatrist.**

shared journey

Notably, such assistance makes this a shared journey of **education** and **discovery**:

- ask questions and be engaged in all levels of your health care;
- identify and explore mitigating social circumstances
  - for example, financial pressures that may impact your ability to eat well, engage in exercise or even afford medications, can be identified and addressed, and
- identification, intervention, support, and monitoring of low mood or depression can receive attention.

There can be multiple barriers to change. The more open you are in helping to identify those barriers, the greater the opportunity is for help to be forthcoming. So, please, speak up.

Change **is** possible. **Education** and **teamwork** are the best places to start.

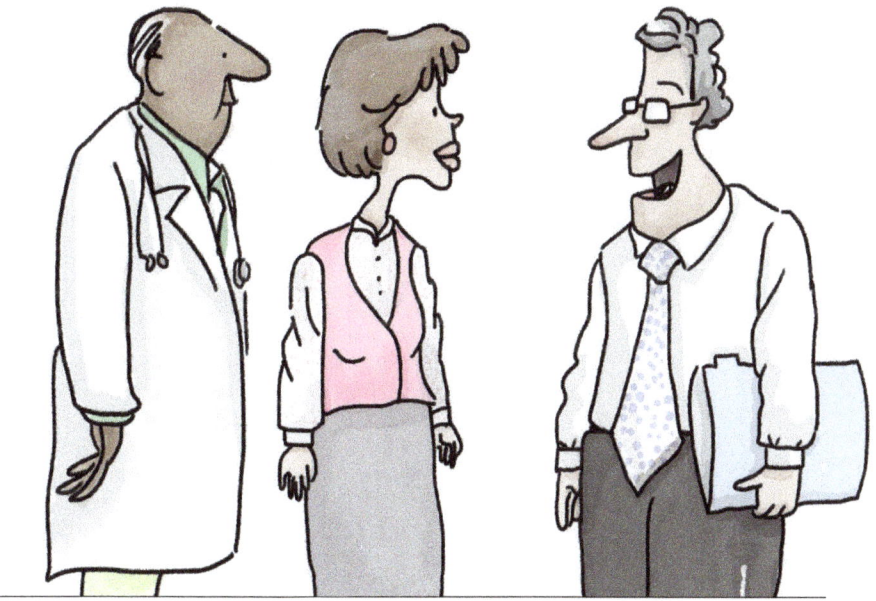

bring your healthcare team together

IMPORTANT POINTS

TEAMWORK

- Plenty of help is readily available.
- Teamwork is better than going it alone.
- ASK!

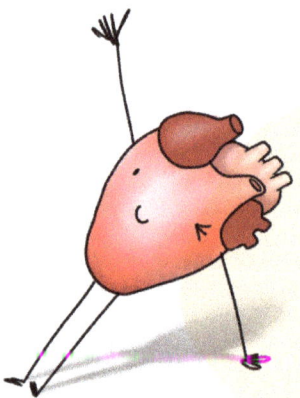

Change is possible, especially:

- ☒ with the help of education
- ☒ through seeking medical advice
- ☒ asking for the support and encouragement of others.

Dan didn't have a heart attack, but he still needed open-heart surgery.

PREVENTION *really is better than cure!*

chapter 15
DAN *DIDN'T* HAVE A HEART ATTACK

Remember Dan from our introduction? That part of his story concluded:

The angiogram itself was quite painless, and the results came back quickly. My worst fears were realised. Not only did I have coronary artery disease (CAD), but it was severe ... severe enough that I was prime for a heart attack and not an insignificant one. My only saving grace was that I was incredibly fortunate to find out through testing rather than my family finding out through an autopsy ... my only option was coronary artery bypass grafting (CABG).

Dan's experience highlights what you are **preventing.**

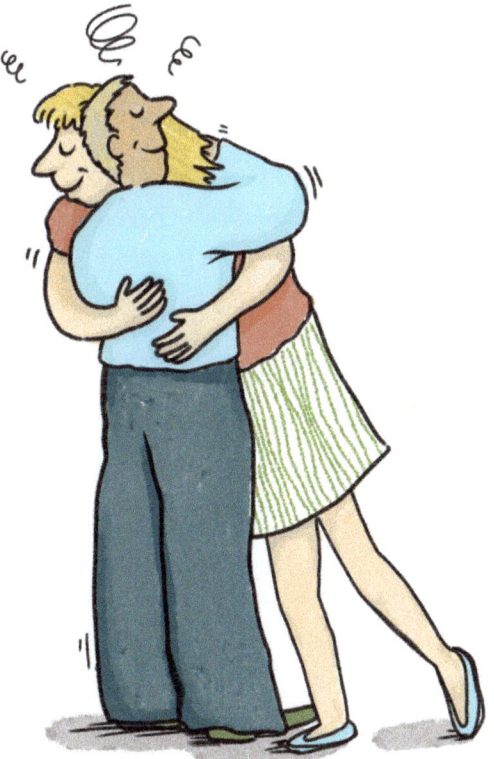

PATIENT'S PERSPECTIVE – DAN (continued)

    Whether it was simply good luck or coincidence, one of Hobart's leading surgeons was at Calvary at the time and was at my bedside shortly after the angiogram results were confirmed. Practising both privately and in the public system, he said he could see me as a patient at the RHH and that I would be classified as a category one patient – for urgent admission. However, I could still expect a 14-28 day waiting period before surgery, and I was warned of the dreaded 'bump' – being scheduled for surgery only to be delayed at short notice due to a more urgent patient.

    I started taking a myriad of medicines to significantly reduce my chances of a heart attack whilst waiting. I was told to rest at home and avoid stressful or physically demanding activities, which I did to the letter because I was petrified. I have – or should I say, had – always taken pride in balanced and strong mental health and a positive outlook, but this left me in an instant.

    Jumping at shadows, the period before surgery was as dark as any of the recovery period. Wearing a heart rate monitor in my watch, I was obsessed with keeping my heart rate under 80, but sometimes my fear alone would trigger a rise that I couldn't control. Perhaps it was the medicines or the fear of the operation, but I was constantly tired and lacked conversation – another first for me.

    I got my call up just over two weeks after the angiogram, and it was such a relief. On reflection, it sounds idiotic to be relieved to be going in for open heart surgery, but I knew it was coming, one way or the other, and the sooner, the better. Unfortunately, COVID restrictions in the hospital were in full force, with only one visitor at a time, for a few hours a day in the afternoon. So, come late afternoon, I entered ward 2D on my own, nervously sitting in the waiting room for directions to my room. As the minutes ticked over to a few hours, I tried reading a book, but the words didn't sink in.

    A text from a medical friend who didn't know I didn't know alerted me to the news that ICU was full and could not take any non-emergency patients. Minutes later, a cardiac anaesthetist arrived to explain the ICU situation. By this time, I was simply numb. I was going home. Forty-five minutes later, one of the ward doctors told me I had been 'bumped'. By then, I felt defeated.

A taxi ride home stands out as one of the lowest points of the entire journey. Physically I was unchanged, but emotionally I was wrecked.

I was fortunate to be rescheduled five days later, being admitted on a Sunday evening.

Check-in went smoothly, and I even lucked into my private room with an ensuite. I'm not sure what I had expected, and I admit that in all my 'research', I hadn't come across or given much thought to where the actual grafts come from to enable the bypass of the arteries. So, a nurse caught me off guard when she told me she would be in before 5 am to complete a full body shave to give the surgeons access to whatever artery and vein they wanted. An artery from the arm and a vein from the leg (with a full-length incision from the elbow to wrist and ankle to knee) were givens, but more might be required depending on what was found. If the magnitude of the operation hadn't dawned on me before this, it certainly had by now. I remember wondering how many arteries and veins would be attacked and what the long-term ramifications might be. Sleep left me.

The morning's shave-down produced a surreal experience – finally being in the pre-surgery phase and locked in for action. No 'bumping' now; it was game on.

They gave me some pre-anaesthetic tablets. The tablets must have been effective because my next memory was a groggy awakening in the ICU and in the care of my very own nurse, whose one role for the day was to look after me.

Only snippets of my stay in the ICU remain. The little button to self-administer pain relief in the form of fentanyl is my most vivid memory. The control was effective. A photo taken by my nurse (at my request) shows a patient with a smile far too large for the procedure just completed. The magic button had a timing switch to avoid overdosing, allowing a small dose at not less than five-minute intervals. A green flashing light would indicate when it was ready, and for no reason I can recall, I became

(continued page 180)

ANSWERING YOUR QUESTIONS

what is coronary artery bypass grafting?

A coronary bypass procedure (coronary artery bypass graft, CABG) uses an artery taken from the chest wall or the wrist, a vein taken from the leg, or sometimes both, to bypass a blockage in one or more of the coronary arteries (the arteries that supply the heart muscle with blood).

Chest wall arteries, particularly the left internal mammary artery (LIMA), are the most used. The radial (arm) artery that supplies blood to the wrist is another common artery used, while the most frequently used vein graft is the saphenous vein taken from the thigh or calf.

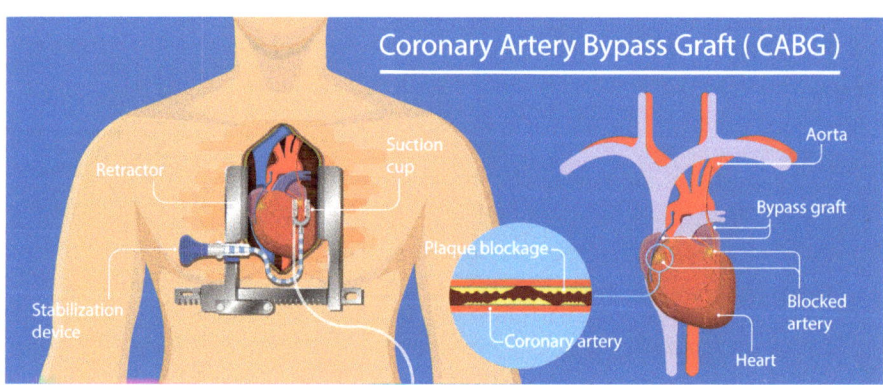

The procedure, done under deep anaesthesia, usually takes between two and three hours depending on the number of grafts involved. Most bypass operations use a mid-line cut in the breastbone (median sternotomy), the ribs are pulled back with special retractors and the heart is placed on bypass using a special heart/lung bypass machine (ECMO, *see page 182*) that oxygenates the blood and pumps the blood while the heart is rested during the surgery. Once the bypass has been performed, the heart is restarted, the circulation begins slowly, and the heart's natural pumping action is gradually restored. Throughout the operation, the patient is on a ventilator.

The patient spends one to two days in the ICU before being transferred to the ward. While in ICU, the patient's natural ventilation is restored.

Pain and discomfort will be experienced post-operatively, in the hospital and at home. Levels are variable and highly personal.

CABG is used for patients with ongoing angina, those not responding to medical treatment, or when stenting is unsuitable for technical reasons. In most situations, it is performed to improve the person's chance of survival. Such situations include narrowing of the left main coronary artery, or where a significant narrowing occurs in all three coronary arteries, particularly if there is some damage to the muscle of the left ventricle.

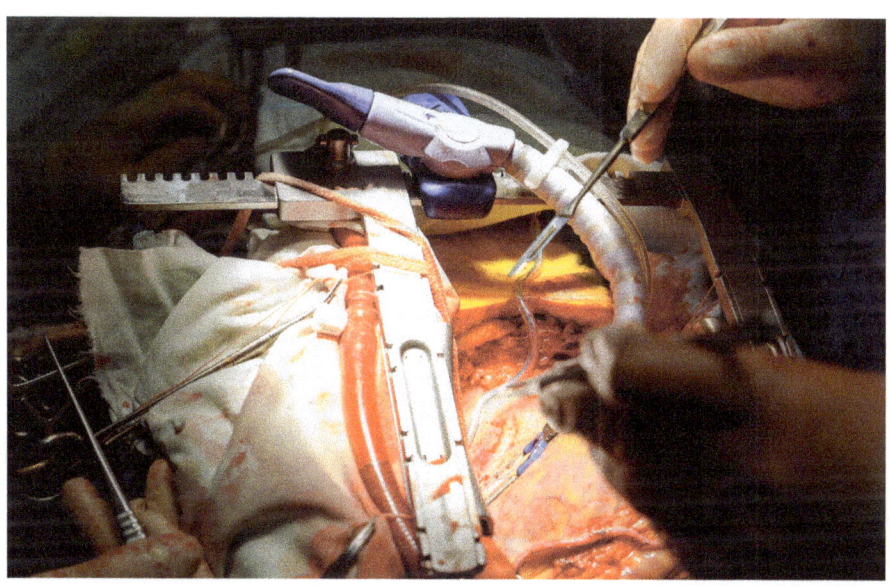

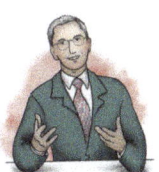

Although it remains a traumatic experience for the patient, bypass surgery is now an extremely efficient procedure that is becoming less invasive.

However, a one-to-two per cent risk of dying from the procedure remains. A similar risk also exists for the person having a stroke or significant heart attack.

Other complications include kidney failure, lung infections such as pneumonia, and blood clots in the legs, which, at times, travel to the lungs.

(from page 177)

engrossed in watching the button and pressing it as soon as I spotted the first flash. In my semi-conscious state, I had a focus, a game to play, and I must have been reasonable at it. I remember the surprise of my nurse when she saw the quantity of fentanyl consumed, and my button was taken off me for a time.

As the day progressed, the discomfort of three tubes inserted into my chest/abdomen (a catheter and two surgery drainage tubes) became more apparent, as did the complete lack of mobility in the chest. I can't recall if it was the same day or the following day when I moved to ward 2D, the cardiac ward at the RHH, but I remember heading to the high-dependency area, as planned, for the initial part of my stay.

Given my age and fitness, I had entered the hospital expecting to excel in recovery and waltz out of the hospital in a matter of days. Instead, for those first few days, I was broken. I couldn't move, and the dim reality of what was ahead was staring me in the face. Katie recalls, on her first visit, a feeling of shock at the sight of me, more from a mental perspective than physically. All lingering pain relief from the anaesthetic had worn off, and even with the fentanyl button back in my possession, both the pain and the discomfort were manifesting. A few hours later, the pain had magnified from uncomfortable to extreme. I had always considered myself to have a high pain tolerance, but this was the next level.

I had hiccups frequently and, on every occurrence, my chest would expand and pressure my wired-up sternum to cause excruciating pain. Efforts to stop the hiccups by holding my breath were ineffective, which was hardly surprising as I had oxygen tubes in my nose to assist my breathing.

A day or two later and I moved to my new room, which, as a positive, was a private room located close to the nurses' station. A negative was its distance from the bathroom and toilet. The small room had the feel of a converted storeroom, but it was home for at least a few days.

I guess things went to plan in the early days, although perhaps not the glossy plan I had in mind.

I was in pain – my green button had been taken away now that I was out of the critical phase.

I had no appetite.

I was immobile.

I was in pain.

I suffered nausea and vomiting throughout the day.

I had to get out of bed daily to sit up in a chair for breakfast and dinner, no mean feat, as moving was brutal, and there was a constant fear that a slip would crack the sternum and cause untold damage.

I was unprepared for the lack of sleep or the semi-conscious nights when I lay in bed

> thinking
>
> not thinking
>
> dreaming
>
> hallucinating, or
>
> simply listening to the monitors at the nurses' station outside the door.

I vividly recall one night lying in bed, unable to sleep, too uncomfortable to move or reach for my earphones, for what appeared to be an eternity – only for a nurse to come in and do the 10 pm observations. Two hours had felt like 10; that night seemed to go on forever. The room was dark, and so was my mind. Thoughts manifested in the wee hours.

I could be dead.

I should be dead.

I'll never surf again.

Why would Katie and the kids want me with such a (perceived) health concern? Even if they did,

> could I be there for them,
>
> would I be ok to work again?

It wasn't a good time.

A few days in, I was asked if I had experienced any bowel movements or stomach rumbling. "Nothing," was my reply, which apparently is not uncommon with the medications I was taking. It was time, I suggested to

A CLOSER LOOK

understanding extra-corporeal membrane oxygenation or ECMO

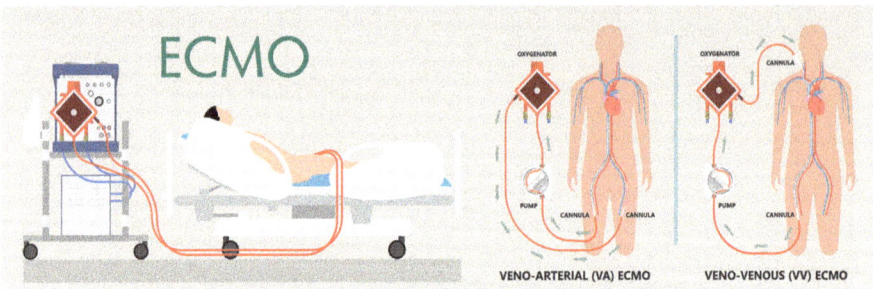

A vital element of many open heart surgeries is 'by-pass', or extra-corporeal membrane oxygenation (ECMO). ECMO comes into play when the heart is stopped so the surgery can be performed.

To keep the patient alive, the blood leaves the body and is treated in a machine that acts as the heart and lungs – outside of the body. After the carbon dioxide-oxygen exchange occurs, the machine pumps the blood back into the body to complete the work of the circulatory system.

ECMO is an extraordinary piece of life-saving technology.

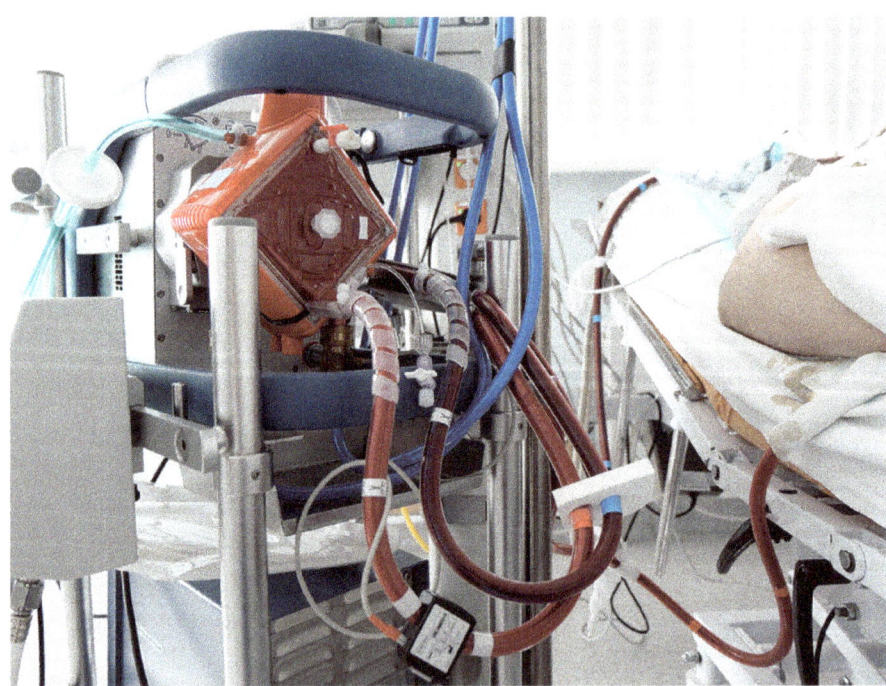

the nurses, so I was provided with some movicol (to ease constipation), which changed the situation not one bit.

The following day, some laxatives were added to the morning tablets – my little cup was now full of a dozen different pills of all sizes and colours – but by lunch there was still no action.

My first session with Chris, the ward physio, was scheduled for the afternoon. He was young and enthusiastic, and he wore nice colourful shirts. One of his roles was getting the patients up and moving following surgery. It was my time. We started with some small steps outside the door of my room, past the nurses' station, where a long corridor awaited us. Towards the end of the corridor, I could see the toilets and showers, probably 30m away, maybe a little more. I was surprised by just how uncomfortable walking was and how little balance I had.

Taking my hand to guide me, Chris was very encouraging and obviously experienced in assisting patients with the first steps post-surgery. A few metres into the journey, he nicely let me know I didn't have to squeeze his hand so tight, but he was wrong. The laxatives must have been working because it was time to go. Actually, it was beyond time to go. A steady stream of liquid was trailing behind me, as well as an odour that was unfavourable to the owner, so I could only guess its effect on those around me, which – being that I was walking past the nurses' station – was many. Chris earned his wages that day as he assisted with increasing pace to seat me on a ward toilet. I had lost bowel control, ended up in nappies, and was embarrassed.

Not the most embarrassed I would be for that day, however. I was fatigued just from this experience, so I was back in bed resting when only a few hours later, I realised my journey with the laxatives was only partially done. On calling for assistance, the nurses quickly opted against a walk back down the corridor and went to fetch what I thought was a wheelchair. Except it wasn't. It looked like one, but it was a chair to sit on, with a toilet seat built in and a pan under it. Filling the pan to the brim, my embarrassment from earlier was quickly erased with a new level that I sincerely hope never to reach again. The nurses were either outstanding workers or exceptional actors. They took it in their stride as if it were a daily occurrence (I hope for their sake it isn't), assisting me back to bed and managing to air the stuffy room to return it to an acceptable level.

I had trouble managing nausea and was vomiting regularly in hospital in the first few days, along with the hiccups. And for an unknown reason, I was also quite down on my oxygen saturation levels, so I was assisted with oxygen for longer than typical for a recovering patient. This surprised me, as I had felt that my fitness levels would be a strength.

Due to COVID, I was only allowed one visitor at a time during a two-hour window. Katie came in daily, which was a godsend, but given the rules, I could not see either of my children whilst in hospital. Not seeing them was a double-edged sword. No doubt I would have gained strength by their presence, but having your children see you when so vulnerable would have been hard on us all.

I had been holding on to the expectation that I could go home after five to six days, and on the sixth morning, I was ready to go. Katie was to pick me up after the 10 am doctor's check, and I was well and truly over my little room. Unfortunately, my body had other plans. Blood tests (which I had daily) revealed a rising trend in several liver counts to levels of concern. So, I was required to stay until further testing showed a path to normality. Whilst obviously of concern, I was again subject to a build-up of expectations suddenly taken away from me, and I didn't like it. I didn't feel any symptoms from the troubled liver count, so mentally, and physically, I felt ready to go home, making it all the harder to remain enthused in my little hospital room.

My only highlight of the extended stay came about one afternoon when Katie negotiated a leave pass from the ward to take me outside for some sun and fresh air in a wheelchair. Our defence will claim that the rules were not black and white, so we made a dash to a nearby shopping arcade where I had a juice in the sun while sitting next to a water fountain. It was magical. It also reinforced the thought that, mentally, it was time to go home.

So, two days later and nine long days after my arrival, my surgeon and I 'negotiated' a departure that morning. The negotiated settlement involved an 'agreement' around daily blood tests (until told otherwise) and a local doctor check-up every second day. The agreement also carried a caveat I might need readmission if things didn't improve.

When Katie picked me up for the journey home, it was such a relief to see the sun. The car ride was uncomfortable but (mostly) manageable.

On the morning I left the hospital, an infection in my right leg developed at the vein removal site. I was given antibiotics, but after a few days at home, it was not improving. The infection became quite severe, to the point I could hardly bear weight on my leg. My doctor took a swab and found that the bug I had was resistant to the antibiotics provided. By the time the results were back from pathology, I was in severe pain even when seated or lying down, and walking was nearly impossible. Perhaps the worst thing about this was the inability to commence walking, which is a key part of the recovery program. I felt I was on hold, losing a valuable opportunity to begin the long path to normality. Fortunately, the new antibiotics began to work, and in a few days, the infection had subsided, and walking was an option.

During my first fortnight at home, sleep did not come easily, and I would wake up around 1 am with severe back pain and shoulder pain. It was debilitating and occurred whenever I lay down for around three to four hours. My only remedy was to sit in my reclining chair and watch a few more episodes of "Breaking Bad". An exceptional series, no doubt, but perhaps not the most uplifting or appropriate series for the 1 am timeslot, post major surgery. I found myself drifting to sleep sometime around 4 am, upright in the chair, until it was morning and Katie would be up to get the kids ready for school.

A chest X-ray showed fluid on the lung, enough to be disappointing (and painful) but not enough to be dangerous. The remedy was to increase my breathing exercises. A vigorous approach to these breathing exercises achieved good results. Combined with improved mobility after overcoming my leg infection, I had turned a corner. It was time to get better.

My liver tests were trending downwards, and for my birthday a few weeks later, I celebrated with a reading in the low range. I was back.

It's incredible how the mind bounces back once small goals are reached. With my liver sorted and no infections, I exercised twice daily, walked the beach with the dogs and appreciated life in general. I believe my moodiness was diminishing (something with which the kids and Katie may or may not agree).

On 31 March, six weeks post-surgery, I was given the go-ahead for slow jogging (with my promise to avoid any trip hazards and the like). I commenced rehabilitation organised by the hospital and set up my program in our home gym based on this. Every day I felt better than the day before.

Finally, on 10 May, 84 days after surgery, I was cleared to return to 'normal' activities, which I celebrated with a trip to Melbourne and a visit to the wave pool with a group of friends. It's safe to say that I wasn't the most mobile or skilled surfer that day, but I'd be surprised if anyone else had a smile as big as mine. I had overcome open heart surgery and had a life in front of me, a life to live.

It's now eight months post-surgery, and I am comfortably living with my 'new normal'. Physically, I am in the realm of 90 per cent pre-surgery fitness, which is close enough. Mentally, I am in an even better place than before. I also possess a life appreciation that can only be experienced when faced with the tangible alternative that all could be taken away.

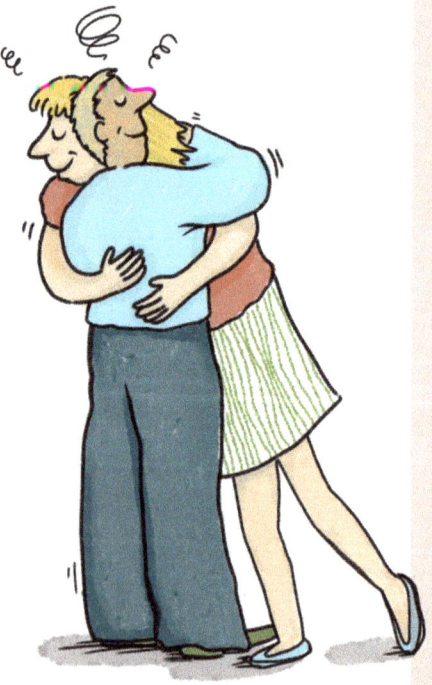

I may never be up for another marathon. Still, today I managed to grind out seven kilometres with Katie and our children. Few people with an angiogram result like mine only months ago could claim such an achievement.

I am one of the lucky ones. I know this and plan to make the most of my second opportunity.

PATIENT'S PERSPECTIVE – RON (continued)

While Dan didn't suffer a heart attack, Ron did.

You will remember that Ron's Monday morning breakfast was interrupted by a heart attack he certainly had **not** put in his diary. Coronary artery bypass surgery was decided as the best treatment because of the number of blocked or imminently blocked arteries. Ron continues.

By first thing on Friday morning, hygienically showered and embarrassingly shaved of pubic hair, I was wheeled into theatre for surgery. I would have liked to have witnessed the surgery, but, of course, I was an unconscious participant.

Around 5 am the next day, I became groggily aware that I was in a bed with tubes in my nose, my neck and my chest as well as a catheter in my penis, a cannula in my arm and wires stuck to my chest. Near the foot of the bed, there was a stand holding a large board behind which stood a nurse making notes on it. I tried to speak and couldn't get any words out. This panicked me but eventually I was able to croak out a question as to what the time was. I was in a high dependency recovery room, but some hours later I was moved to the cardiac intensive care unit. About a day later (I am not certain of the timing) I was moved into the general cardiac ward.

The first few days after my heart surgery were very uncomfortable. In fact, I felt the epitome of the saying 'death warmed up'. I was on pain killers, including oxycodone, and other medications. As best I remember, they included esomeprazole, metoprolol, amlodipine, heparin, atorvastatin, potassium and magnesium, and a laxative. The latter did not have much effect as I remained constipated for about five days.

To prevent opening the chest wound and to allow the bones to knit together, the requirement not to use my arms to

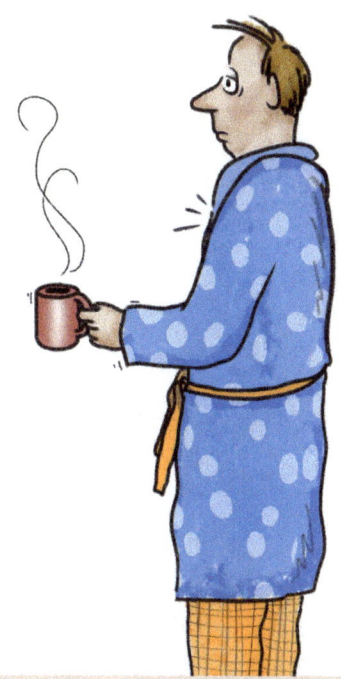

brace and turn over in bed made it difficult to sleep. To sit up or get out of bed, I had to use a cord attached to the end of the bed to pull myself upright, holding my arms tight against my body, then carefully swing my legs over the side of the bed. Of course, every hour or two I was disturbed for the delivery of medication, taking of blood pressure, and other disruptions. Getting a good night's sleep in hospital proved to be impossible.

To help clear the lungs, I was required periodically to hold a folded towel with my arms crossed across my chest, inhale deeply for a few breaths then cough. This was painful to do, and it took some will on my part to comply. On the other hand, fear of involuntary coughing damaging my chest wound meant most of the time I hugged that folded towel like a security blanket. I regularly used a mask to breath vapor to help my lungs rehydrate.

For the first few days I was attached to a drip into my arm and monitoring pads attached to my torso connected to a portable relay device. To move from the bed, I needed to wheel the drip stand and carry the monitoring device attached to the monitoring pads. In a way I was glad to be constipated as it lessened the number of times I had to juggle getting out of bed and moving. Since I couldn't twist sideways in bed to reach the side tables, it was a frustration that nurses and visitors would place or move water, food, and other items to them, requiring me to make the laborious effort to get out of bed to reach things. When I was finally allowed to shower, doing so without getting the monitoring device wet was a real challenge.

Then, I began to develop a bed sore. I also developed a sore area in the back of the calf of my left leg (from which a vein had been extracted for

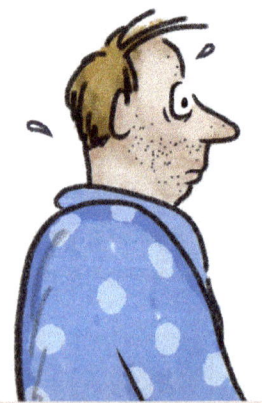

my bypass surgery). I reported this a couple of times, but the Registrar dismissed this as being of no concern. However, when the surgeon visited me on his rounds, and I mentioned the sore area, he ordered an ultrasound. To the apparent surprise of the medical staff, given the amount of anti-clotting medications I was receiving, the ultrasound identified that I had a deep vein thrombosis (DVT) in my calf.

A problem developed with the cannula and my arm became quite painful and seeped blood, but no-one seemed to want to take responsibility for it.

I began to feel a sense of disbelief and despair at my situation. Although it wasn't something I had dwelt on consciously, I realised I had a strong self-image of being a healthy person. My heart attack and heart surgery completely undermined that.

Until this, I had never taken more medications than a couple of tablets for an occasional headache. Now I was on multiple medications and told that some of them I would need to take for the rest of my life. Getting off as many of these medications became a bit of a focus for me and it took about 18 months before I gave up my concerns and came to accept my new reality.

I was encouraged to get up and walk as soon as possible and I began to walk a circuit around the ward as I recovered my strength. Just before I was due to be discharged, I was given a CT scan which revealed considerable fluid in my lungs. My discharge was delayed so that my lungs could be drained by inserting a drain in my back through my lower ribs on my left side. Nurses warned me that this would be painful and gave me two oxycodone a short time before the procedure. I was given local anaesthetic at the site of the insertion and felt little pain at that juncture.

However, once the drain was through into my lungs, I experienced the most severe pain I had ever experienced. Literally, the excruciating pain only hurt if I breathed. I began sweating, crying and dreaded each breath. The nurses gave me another two oxycodone, and within half an hour the pain gradually eased. I entered a relaxed drug induced state, and that night had the best and only good sleep I had during my hospitalisation. No wonder opioids so easily capture people to addiction.

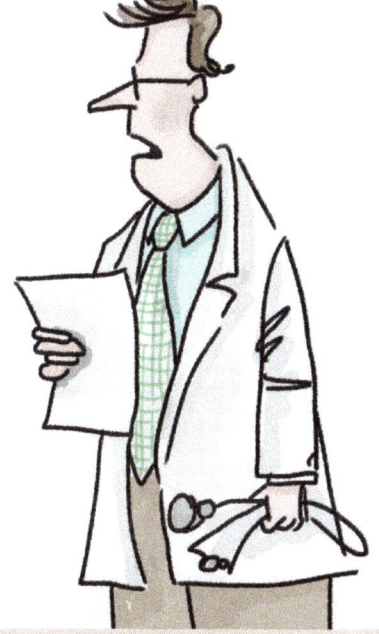

Thirteen days after admission, Ron went home – with a cocktail of prescribed drugs and an instruction sheet on when to take them.

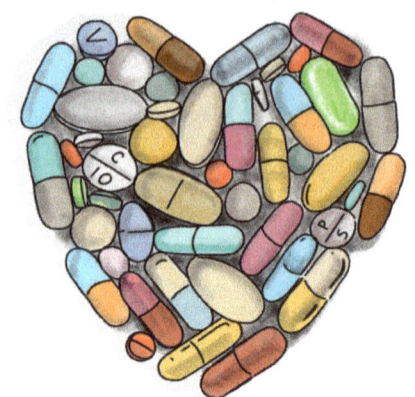

Unfortunately, his problems continued.

He needed a new GP. His long-time GP had closed his practice and the default practice could not see him for two weeks when he needed an appointment for the day after discharge.

Movement remained limited.

Sharp and intense pain in his right shoulder and down his right arm resulted in a trip to Emergency, but nothing was discovered, even after an ultrasound later at Calvary Hospital.

A disturbing and confusing sequence of events involving several specialists, another trip to Emergency and emerging stomach issues resulted in Ron asking to be referred to a private cardiologist for ongoing monitoring and advice.

Ron concludes,

I continue living as healthily as I can.

Nevertheless, I live with a heightened sense of my mortality, that awareness more pronounced when I experience the occasional twinges of pain or discomfort in my chest. At such times, I wonder, Is my heart about to suffer another attack? Will this be the end game?

To be prepared, I have done the necessary organisational things such as updating my will, setting up power of attorney, organising finances and other matters so as not to leave behind too much of a mess for others to clean up.

Otherwise, I just try to get on with life.

IMPORTANT POINTS

DAN *DIDN'T* HAVE A HEART ATTACK

- Open heart surgery is a physically, emotionally and mentally traumatic experience.
- Coronary artery bypass grafting is a life-saving surgical procedure used to treat coronary heart disease.
- Extra-corporeal membrane oxygenation (ECMO) is an extraordinary piece of life-saving technology that keeps the patient alive while the heart is stopped for surgery.
- And Ron DID have a heart attack. Either way, the journey is challenging and personal.

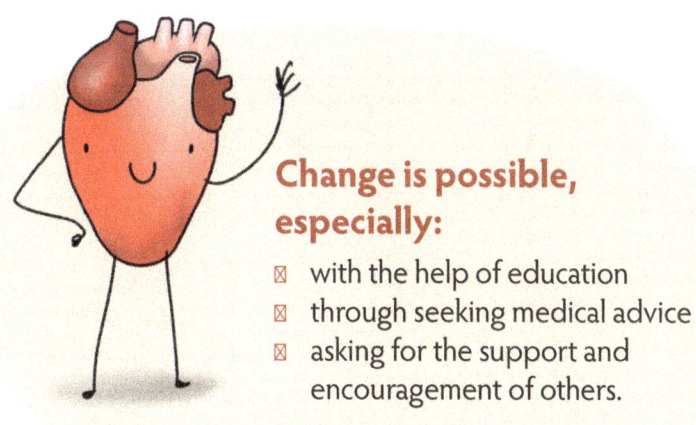

Change is possible, especially:
- ☒ with the help of education
- ☒ through seeking medical advice
- ☒ asking for the support and encouragement of others.

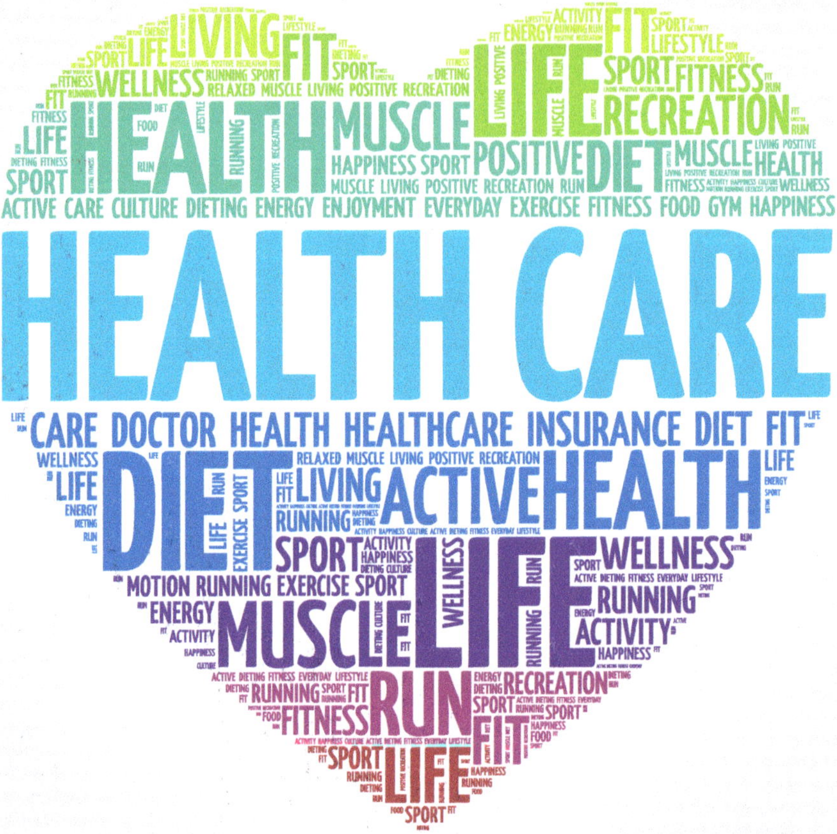

New opportunities for others to live emerge from death.

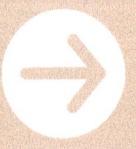

epilogue
LIFE AFTER DEATH

An Australian former world-class ironman surf lifesaving and ocean paddling champion Guy Leech has taken on a new life saving role[82] since the sudden death of a best mate while paddling off a Sydney beach one morning.

"I always loved the fitness aspect of being an ironman," Guy told me (WB) in a podcast conversation for my Healthy Heart Network (16 January 2022, episode 212[83]). So, when his competitive days were over, he became a trainer.

One morning in 2016, he had a fitness class of 25 on a Sydney beach when one of them, Chucky, suffered a sudden cardiac arrest (SCA).

"He was one of my best mates, this guy, and he dropped at the end of the session.

"My training from the surf club days jumped in, and we made sure we rang 000. The ambulance was on the way, and I started resuscitating him. The ambulance took about 13-14 minutes to turn up. I kept resuscitating him and didn't get a result. (It) wasn't just me pumping his chest, trying to get him back. It was the other 24 people there – all mates with him as well, watching it. It was just, just an horrific situation."

The sudden cardiac arrest (SCA), which caused Chucky's collapse, is an electrical issue with the heart; it is not a heart attack[84] as we have been discussing throughout this book, although SCA can be a consequence of a heart attack, as it was in this case. Today (as you are reading this page), there will be close to 100 Aussies who drop dead from an electrical issue with their heart.

The significance of this episode in this epilogue is what Guy told me next.

"There were 100 people in my group: fit, predominantly males, 40-70 years of age. They were probably in the top one per cent in health and wellness from a fitness, eating, and lifestyle point of view.

"After Chucky passed away, I said to them, *You've got 12 weeks to go and get your heart checked. Get a referral to a cardiologist and get checked out because we don't want to be doing this again. We want to know what's going on inside our bodies,* which most of them didn't know.

"And so, 100 fit, healthy Aussies from the age of 40-70 went for a check-up.

"Five of them had to have stents put in straight away.

"One had two put in. He was the 40-year-old who was the fittest in the group and was about to represent Australia two weeks later in America, in a five-hour race, running, swimming, paddling, and cycling.

"Fifteen others had to go on medication."

Prevention! Prevention! Prevention!

These are not random statistics. These were 100 fit, healthy ordinary Australians who work out on a typical day.

Prevention! Prevention! Prevention!

As you will have gleaned from this book, from my previous books and all my work on social media, and through the Healthy Heart Network, **my passion is prevention** – preventing that first heart episode, and if I'm too late for that, then preventing subsequent events.

Let's recap some figures – move over COVID:

- More than 18,600 Australians die yearly from heart disease, 51 people a day or one person every 28 minutes.
- In the United States, 640,000 Americans die from heart disease every year or more than 1750 a day. One person has a heart attack every 40 seconds.

These figures are staggering.

Too regularly, we see the pain, suffering and grief caused by heart disease, and our specific interest in this book, heart attack. The financial, mental, physical and emotional costs are enormous, impacting beyond the immediate sufferer to family, friends, and colleagues.

Simple lifestyle tweaks can markedly reduce your risk.

Being ahead of the game by knowing your coronary artery calcium score could save your life.

Our deep desire, always, is to provide you with information that can help you be involved in your destiny and give yourself the best chance at a healthy life. So, it is now over to you.

Our ongoing hope is that you will live as well as possible for as long as possible.

Good health.

Warrick Bishop
Hobart, Tasmania, Australia

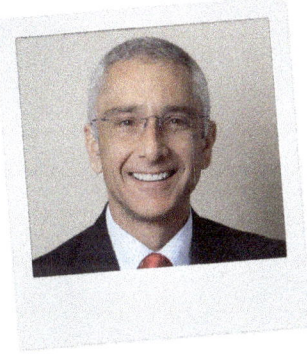

Karam Kostner
Brisbane, Queensland, Australia

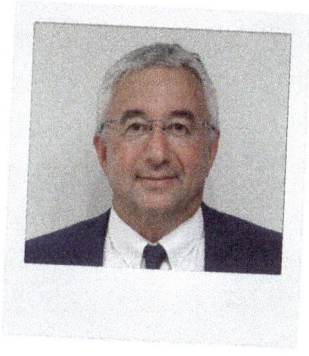

---

82   *Heart 180 (https://heart180.com.au/) Also see appendix 4, page 203*

83   *Healthy Heart Network podcast episode 212 https://drwarrickbishop.com/s/guy*

84   *A heart attack is a consequence of clogged or blocked arteries; the person continues to breathe and may or may not collapse. A sudden cardiac arrest is an electrical issue that can happen to anyone at any time but most commonly is triggered by a heart attack. The heart stops pumping, and the person stops breathing and collapses. Quickly restarting the heart (by cardiac pulmonary resuscitation [CPR] and/or defibrillation) is the person's only chance of survival.*

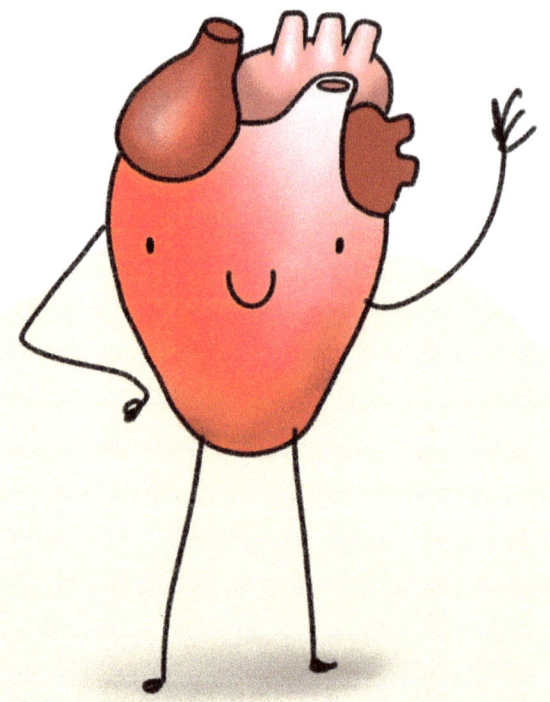

Change is possible, especially:
- with the help of education
- through seeking medical advice
- asking for the support and encouragement of others.

APPENDICES

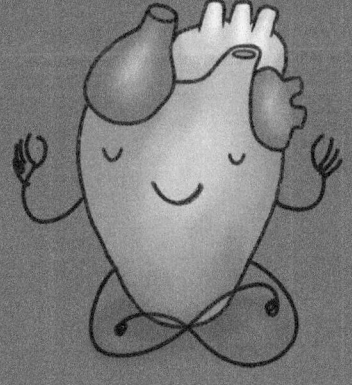

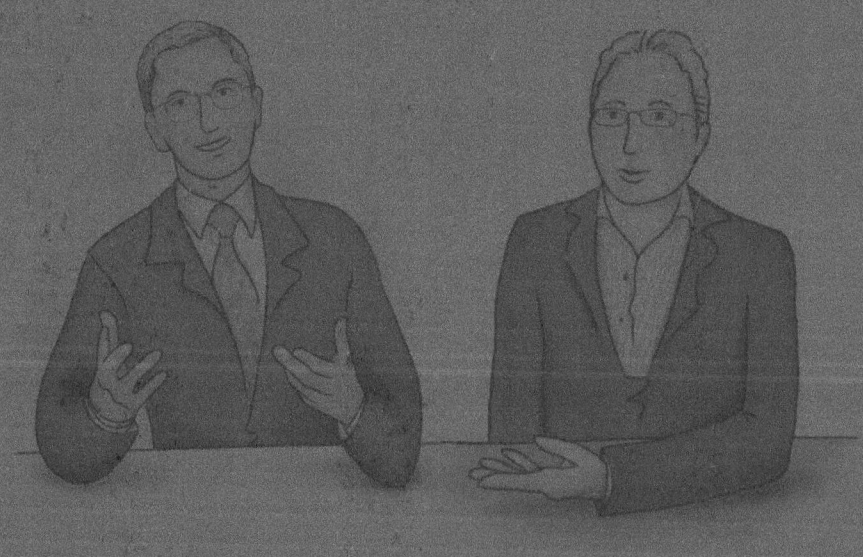

appendix 1
WILL YOU RECOGNISE YOUR HEART ATTACK?

Will you recognise your heart attack?
Warning Signs Action Plan

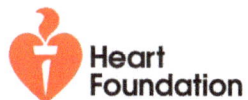

Do you feel any
pain · pressure · heaviness · tightness

In one or more of your
chest · neck · jaw · arm/s · back · shoulder/s

You may also feel
nauseous · a cold sweat · dizzy · short of breath

Yes

1 STOP and rest now

2 TALK tell someone how you feel

If you take angina medicine
- Take a dose of your medicine.
- Wait 5 minutes. Still have symptoms? Take another dose of your medicine.
- Wait 5 minutes. Symptoms won't go away?

Are your symptoms severe or getting worse? **or** Have your symptoms lasted 10 minutes?

Yes

3 CALL 000 Triple Zero
and chew 300mg aspirin, unless you have an allergy to aspirin or your doctor has told you not to take it

- Ask for an ambulance.
- Don't hang up.
- Wait for the operator's instructions.

© 2019 National Heart Foundation of Australia ABN 98 008 419 761. HH-PWS-002.1.0119

appendix 2
SOBERING STATISTICS[85]

Cardiovascular disease (CVD) is an umbrella term that includes heart, stroke, and blood vessel diseases and is one of Australia's largest health problems.

Heart disease is the broad term for conditions that affect the structure and function of the heart muscle. Issues include coronary heart disease, heart failure, valve disease, arrhythmias, congenital heart defects, weakened heart muscle and inflammation.

CORONARY HEART DISEASE (CHD) occurs when the coronary arteries narrow or block because of plaque build-up. **CHD includes heart attack (acute myocardial infarction) and all consequences associated with 'bad' arteries.** As detailed throughout this book, CHD is largely preventable as many of its risk factors are modifiable.

Even so, **CHD is the leading single cause of disease burden and death in Australia**.

In 2021, CHD accounted for 17,300 deaths (AIHW 2023c). This represented 10% of all deaths and 41% of cardiovascular disease deaths. **Thirty-eight per cent (6500) of CHD deaths resulted from a heart attack**.

In 2020-21, an estimated 571,000 Australians aged 18 and over (2.9% of the adult population) were living with CHD, based on self-reported data from the Australian Bureau of Statistics 2020-21 National Health Survey (ABS 2022). The prevalence of CHD increases rapidly with age, affecting around 1 in 9 (11%) of adults aged 75 and over.

In 2020, an estimated **56,700 people** aged 25 and over had **an acute coronary event** as either a heart attack or unstable angina – **around 155 events every day**. Of these, **6900 (12%) were fatal**.

In 2023, CHD was the leading specific cause of burden in Australia, with 305,000 years of healthy life lost – equivalent to 11.5 disability-adjusted life years (DALY) per 1000 population. (DALY is a measure of the overall disease burden, representing the number of healthy years lost due to illness, disability, or premature death.) The burden was twice as high in males, at

206,000 DALY, as in females (99,000 DALY). It increased rapidly from age 45 onwards – from 6.5 DALY per 1000 among people aged 45–49, to 190 per 1000 among people aged 95–99 (AIHW 2023a).

CHD accounted for 5.4% of the total burden of disease in Australia. It comprised 9.1% of the fatal burden and 2.2% of the non-fatal burden.

In 2020–21, the estimated expenditure on CHD was $2.5 billion. The greatest cost was due to private hospital services, and public hospital admitted patient services ($957.9 million and $915.8 million, respectively). The estimated Pharmaceutical Benefits Scheme (PBS) expenditure related to CHD was $156.2 million (AIHW 2023b).

As a result of the substantial impact of CHD on the Australian population, a national Strategic Action Plan for Heart Disease and Stroke has been developed. The action plan aims to reflect priorities and identify implementable actions to reduce the impact of CHD in the community.

The CHD death rate is falling. This decline has been attributed to a combination of factors, including reductions in some risk factor levels, better treatment and care, and improved secondary prevention (ABS 2018).

---

85   *Heart, stroke and vascular disease: Australian facts; Australian Institute of Health and Welfare (14 December 2023)*

https://www.aihw.gov.au/reports/heart-stroke-vascular-disease/hsvd-facts/contents/summary-of-coronary-heart-disease-and-stroke/coronary-heart-disease

other relevant Australian and global statistics are available at sites including

the Australian figures in this appendix are taken from the Heart Foundation website, which were sourced from the Australian Bureau of Statistics and the Australian Institute of Health and Welfare 2020, National Hospital Morbidity Database (NHMD)

cardiovascular disease:
www.heartfoundation.org.au/bundles/for-professionals/key-stats-cardiovascular-disease

heart disease:
www.heartfoundation.org.au/bundles/for-professionals/australia-heart-disease-statistics

coronary heart disease:
www.heartfoundation.org.au/bundles/for-professionals/coronary-heart-disease-key-stats

heart attack:
www.heartfoundation.org.au/bundles/for-professionals/coronary-heart-disease-key-stats

risk factors of cardiovascular disease:
www.heartfoundation.org.au/bundles/for-professionals/key-statistics-risk-factors-for-heart-disease

the global figures are taken from World Health Organization, FAQ sheet 11 June 2021
www.who.int/news-room/fact-sheets/detail/cardiovascular-diseases-(cvds)

appendix 3
SWAP[86] THIS FOR THAT

potato crisps	unsalted nuts and seeds
	air popped popcorn – try adding spices or chilli flakes instead of salt and butter
hot chips	home-made sweet potato wedges (toss wedges of sweet potato with olive oil and bake @180oC for 20-30 minutes)
sweet biscuits and cakes	home-made versions *see recipes at* www.heartfoundation.org.au/recipes/category/baking
fruit yoghurt or ice cream	natural yoghurt with added fresh or frozen berries
ham sandwich	cheese and salad sandwich on wholemeal bread
meat pie	chicken and salad wrap
cream cheese, cheese spread, cheese sticks	mozzarella, edam, cheddar, cottage and Swiss cheese
salt	herbs, spices, pepper, garlic, chilli, or ginger
soft drinks, fruit juice or cordial	water, mineral water, or sparkling water – try adding lemon, lime or orange slices to flavour the water without using sugar

---

86 *The Heart Foundation website https://www.heartfoundation.org.au/getmedia/d9ca1d68-fdb3-4efe-9716-5dfeb2802c1e/Eating-well-to-protect-your-heart.pdf*

appendix 4
SURVIVING THE ODDS: DEFIBRILLATORS SAVE LIVES

Sudden cardiac death — also sudden cardiac arrest and unexplained cardiac death — is one of the biggest killers of Australians under 50 and is five times more likely to affect men. The primary cause of SCD in adults 35 and over is coronary heart disease. In younger people (under 35) it is congenital heart conditions and heart rhythm disorders. Many of the younger people affected by SCD are generally regarded as being fit and healthy. Little information exists on why the problem occurs. In Australia, the rates of SCD in people aged under 35 years are thought to be one in 30,000[87], and in middle-aged people is it likely to be a least twice this figure[88].

Defibrillation is effective in over 90 per cent of cases if applied within one minute, but ineffective in over 90 per cent if applied 10 minutes later, even if cardio-pulmonary resuscitation (CPR) is performed[89].

'WHAT IF?' LEADS TO HEART 180

The morning Chucky died (*see page 193*) changed Guy Leech's life irrevocably.

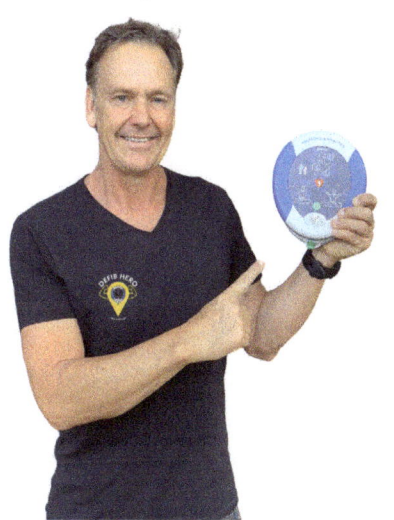

He discovered that morning that CPR (cardio-pulmonary resuscitation) – even good CPR he had learnt during his surf lifesaving days – was not enough to restart heart once it had gone into arrhythmia and stopped.

Following Chucky's death, Guy founded the national company Heart 180 distribute two world-leading brands of defibrillators. Heart 180's mission is to have a defibrillator within 180 seconds of every Australian.

When a person has a sudden cardiac arrest (SCA), an electrical malfunction causes the heart to stop beating. As a result, the person effectively 'drops dead'. However, a window of opportunity lasting 180 seconds – three minutes – gives the person the best chance of breathing again.

That summer experience, in which all the correct procedures were followed but were not enough, forced Guy to rethink his life's purpose and to question what he was doing professionally and personally.

What if there had a defibrillator in the car?

What if the café nearby had had a defibrillator?

What if one of my kids or my wife was to suffer a sudden cardiac arrest?

Where is the nearest defibrillator now?

In Australia, about 30,000 people suffer a sudden cardiac arrest each year – 600 people a week – including kids, teenagers, and fit adults. Less than 10 per cent – thought to be closer to six per cent – of those people survive.

The chance of survival increases to 70 per cent when an onlooker uses a defibrillator within three minutes of the collapse.

That 180 seconds can be the difference between life and death.

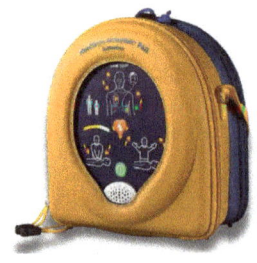

Sudden cardiac arrest can strike anyone at any time. Anyone can use a defibrillator, even without training, although Heart 180 recommends training.

further information: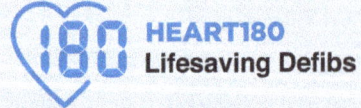

Heart 180
https://drwarrickbishop.com/s/heart180

Healthy Heart Network
https://healthyheartnetwork.com/survey/show/61

https://drwarrickbishop.com/s/guy

SECOND CHANCE[90] BRINGS NEW PASSION

Greg Page AM is an Australian singer, musician, and actor who was a founding member, the lead singer and the original Yellow Wiggle in the internationally successful phenomenon, The Wiggles, an Australian children's entertainment band.

At the end of an Original Wiggles, adults-only, concert held in January 2020 to raise funds for victims of the devastating bushfires of the 2019-2020 Australian summer, Greg went into cardiac arrest at the end of the concert and 'died' on stage. Thanks to the quick action of several people and that the concert venue had a defibrillator, he survived.

 The following exchange is from Dr Bishop's Healthy Heart Network's podcasts #163, 164. The interview also features in Dr Bishop's previous book, *Cardiac Rehabilitation Explained* (2023).

WB You sound very much like an average 40-something-year-old bloke who'd put on a bit of weight then lost a bit of weight. Maybe could have eaten a bit better, but you did a bit of exercise. You didn't have much in the way of a family history as a flag. Your cholesterol was a bit on the high side, but not catastrophically high. From what you described, there's no major flag, Greg, and that really leads us on to the guts of this interview, which is the event that you had. I heard it on the news, as I guess many people did. Can you walk me through what happened?

G *There's not a lot I can remember to be honest.*

So, the 17th of January was the day after my 48th birthday. We had this performance to do for The Wiggles. I was very conscious that I had to do a show; we hadn't done a show in some time. So, I was conscious about my physical fitness. I'd been walking and exercising, staying relatively fit. I don't remember a lot about the day itself, nor the show... But one of the things I can remember is lying on the ground after I'd collapsed – you know, going into cardiac arrest.

With the benefit of hindsight, I can tell everybody that what happened physiologically inside my body was a clot had formed in my LAD, my left anterior descending artery, in my heart and blocked off that artery. Apparently 100 per cent. And almost immediately, I would say, I went into cardiac arrest.

*I don't remember any warning signs. I don't remember feeling heavy in the chest or any pain or any shortness of breath, other than what I would normally experience during a Wiggles' show when you're being physically active and exerting yourself. I was out of breath, and that's what I can remember. I don't remember the moment of collapsing, but I do remember lying on the floor, looking up at the ceiling, and struggling to breathe. I remember thinking, Gosh, I'm **so** out of breath. I'm **so** exhausted after that show, but I didn't think that that could have been my last few breaths on this earth.*

WB Was that memory – of you lying on the floor looking up – after you had been resuscitated, Greg?

G I think that was before I passed out. It was like, the last few breaths I was taking. Luckily, people around me recognised that I was in cardiac arrest or that I needed CPR (cardio-pulmonary resuscitation) and they jumped straight onto it. Called triple zero, of course, and then straight into the CPR. So, I'm very, very fortunate.

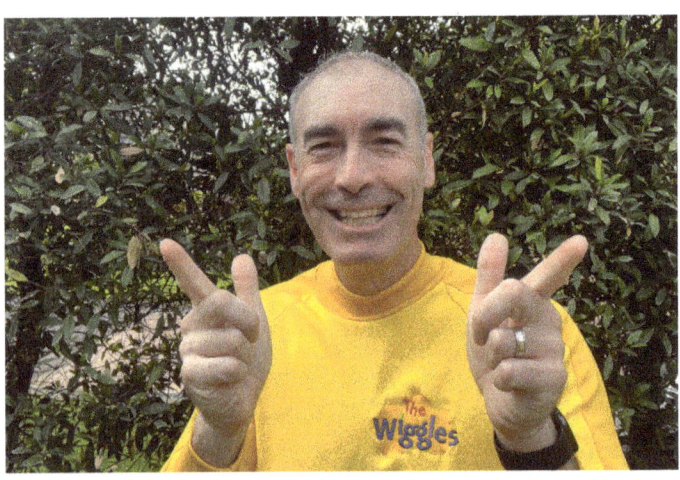

Greg Page as a very active Yellow Wiggle, when he thought he was fit and healthy.

further on in the interview ...

G   *Yeah, look, it is a big thing. I view every day now as a bonus, and I have a mission. I'm still doing the other things that I used to do. That is, I'm still working in the children's entertainment field and trying to do what I can to produce shows for children.* **But I'm now on a mission** *to educate older people as well, about heart disease and cardiac arrest, and the difference between cardiac arrest and heart attack, and CPR (cardio-pulmonary resuscitation) and AED (automated external defibrillator).*

Given that stat about how many people survive a cardiac arrest and the fact that it is so low, I think we've got a long way to go in terms of educating people about response to cardiac arrest and improving those outcomes for people. So, **more people knowing CPR, having more AEDs available and knowing where they are and how to use them** *– there's a big mission there for me that I really feel compelled to be contributing towards.*

WB   For those (reading) who are not up with the abbreviated terms, what are they, Greg?

G   *CPR stands for cardio-pulmonary resuscitation, and AED stands for automated external defibrillator.*

And so, one of the big things about AEDs, or those defibrillators, that people probably don't understand, is that you don't need to be medically qualified or certified to use one to save a life. On the night that I needed to be shocked with an AED, there was a nurse there, but any one of those bystanders could have used that AED to shock my heart back into a normal rhythm. And that's what people need to know – you can't hurt somebody by using an AED because it will not shock somebody who doesn't need to be shocked. The pads that you place on the chest of the patient will determine if that patient needs to be shocked. And the AED talks to you and tells you what to do. It will only say push the shock button if it needs to deliver a shock to that patient. And you, as the user of the device, can't be harmed, either.

and further on ...

G   *Live every day as if it could be last because you just don't know. At the same time, live it as if you don't want it to be your last. Life is an incredible gift and I absolutely love life... So, if you want to live an amazing life, you can do it. Live it today because there might not be tomorrow. If there is a tomorrow, make sure it's the best it can be.*

So, act now and get your heart checked out. Don't have that 1-in-10 chance of surviving a cardiac arrest. That's the only message I would say. Take care of yourself, everybody.

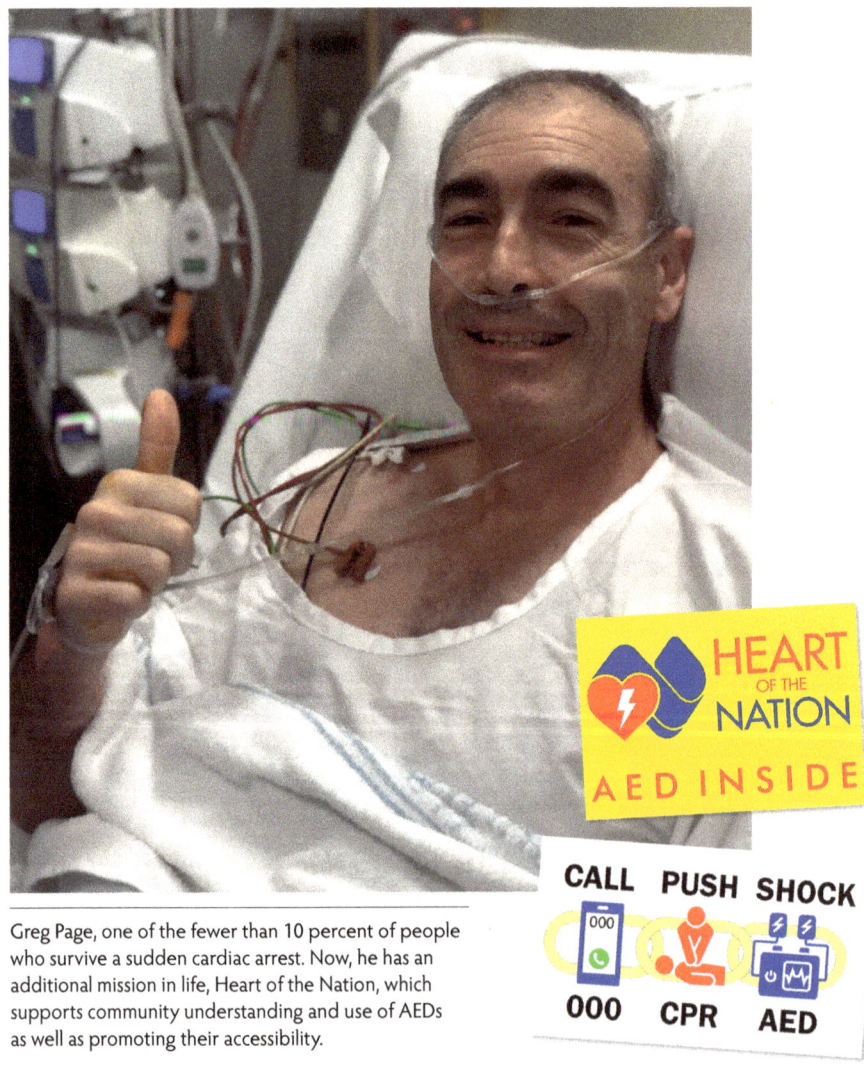

Greg Page, one of the fewer than 10 percent of people who survive a sudden cardiac arrest. Now, he has an additional mission in life, Heart of the Nation, which supports community understanding and use of AEDs as well as promoting their accessibility.

Heart of the Nation

As a result of his cardiac arrest, Greg has a new mission in life, an initiative called Heart of the Nation. He explains:

"I believe there is a lack of understanding about AEDs in the community and where you can find them if one is needed. Heart of the Nation is like that Australian Made program with the little logo that goes on Australian-made products."

Any company, business, community group that has an AED on site can become a member of Heart of the Nation. An extensive website provides detailed information about Heart of the Nation initiatives such as its community, business and medical associations, the Great Aussie AED Hunt, the CPR Pushathon and its AED locator app.

"More people need to know about AEDs and know where to find one should a life be endangered. I want to promote that because I've been the beneficiary of an AED working well and I want other people to benefit the same way."

further information:

Heart of the Nation
https://www.heartofthenation.com.au/

Chain of Survival
https://www.heartofthenation.com.au/chain-of-survival

Healthy Heart Network
https://drwarrickbishop.com/s/greg

---

87 Semsarian et al. New England Journal of Medicine 2016
88 https://baker.edu.au/health-hub/sudden-cardiac-death
89 O'Rourke, M.F (2010) Reality of Out of Hospital Cardiac Arrest, BMJ Journals.
90 Greg Page, Healthy Heart Network podcasts # 163, 164; Beating the Odds, Warrick Bishop, Alistair Begg, Cardiac Rehabilitation Explained, pp 219-232 (2023)

ACCESS YOUR BOOK BONUSES

Unlock the full potential of your reading experience with exclusive access to our special book bonuses. Dive deeper into the vital topic of heart health with our carefully curated selection of bonus materials designed to complement your journey through the pages with expert and patient interviews and bonus videos, including TEDx talks, Heart Attacks are Preventable! and Prevention is Better Than Cure mini-courses.

podcast interviews

- Darren Lehmann, *international cricketer*: https://drwarrickbishop.com/s/darren

- Greg Page, *international entertainer*: https://drwarrickbishop.com/s/greg

- Ralf Ilchef, *liaison psychiatrist*: https://drwarrickbishop.com/s/ralf

- Robert Zecchin, *cardiac rehabilitation clinician-researcher*: https://drwarrickbishop.com/s/rob

other resources

- Weight Loss Course: https://drwarrickbishop.com/s/tfbsg

- Atrial Fibrillation Kit: https://drwarrickbishop.com/s/afkit

- Healthy Heart Network Membership: https://healthyheartnetwork.com

- Heart Attacks are Preventable Webinar: https://healthyheartnetwork.com

- How Healthy is Your Heart, Really? https://drwarrickbishop.com/s/vhc

- Download our free Mobile App: https://healthyheartnetwork.com/page/mobile

other books by Dr Warrick Bishop

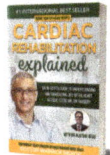
Cardiac Rehabilitation Explained: is a must read for anyone who has recently experienced a cardiac event, such as a heart attack, stenting, or cardiac surgery. In explaining the importance of cardiac rehabilitation, this comprehensive guide provides a thorough understanding of the causes, treatments available, and the steps individuals can take to recover or improve their cardiovascular health, thus also making this book a powerful preventative tool for those who wish, at any age, to be proactive about their health (with Dr Alistair Begg).

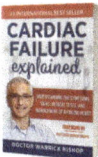
Cardiac Failure Explained: a complete guide to understanding and managing heart failure, covering everything from the causes and symptoms of heart failure to the latest treatment options available.

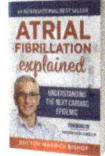
Atrial Fibrillation Explained: a comprehensive guide that provides an easy-to-understand overview of atrial fibrillation, covering its causes, symptoms, and treatment options.

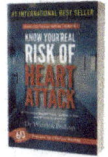
Know Your Real Risk of Heart Attack: explains the various risk factors that contribute to heart disease and provides practical advice on how to reduce your risk, making it an excellent resource for anyone looking to take control of their heart health.

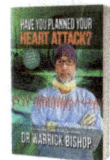
Have You Planned Your Heart Attack?: offers a balanced and referenced discussion of coronary risk assessment using modern technology, specifically, CT scans to evaluate the health of coronary arteries.

https://drwarrickbishop.com/s/books

REFERENCES

10 Commandments of Heart Health Explained has been informed by

AHA Guidelines

24 Bulletin

Living dangerously: Australians with multiple risk factors for cardiovascular disease; Bulletin, Issue 24, February 2005; Australian Institute of Health and Wealth (Australian Government)

books, text:

Begg, Alistair; *What's Wrong with My Heart?* (unpublished text)

Begg, Alistair, Bishop, Warrick; *Cardiac Rehabilitation Explained* (2023)

Bishop, Warrick; *Have You Planned Your Heart Attack?* (2016)

Bishop, Warrick; *Atrial Fibrillation Explained* (2019)

Bishop, Warrick; *Cardiac Failure Explained* (2020)

websites:

American Heart Association	https://www.heart.org/
Australian Institute of Health and Welfare	https://www.aihw.gov.au/
Diabetes Australia	http://www.diabetesaustralia.com.au/
Heart Foundation (Australia)	https://www.heartfoundation.org
Heart Research Institute (Australia)	https://www.hri.org.au
National Alcohol and Other Drug Hotline	https://www.health.gov.au/contacts/national-alcohol-and-other-drug-hotline
National Health and Medical Research Council (NHMRC, Australia)	https://www.nhmrc.gov.au/
National Heart, Lung and Blood Institute	https://www.nhlbi.nih.gov/
National Library of Medicine (National Centre for Biotechnology Information)	https://www.ncbi.nlm.nih.gov/
ResearchGate	https://www.researchgate.net/
The Lancet	https://www.thelancet.com/
The New England Journal of Medicine	https://www.nejm.org/
World Economic Forum	https://www.weforum.org/
World Health Organization	https://www.who.int/

GLOSSARY

A

acute coronary syndrome (ACS)
describes a range of conditions resulting from reduced blood flow to the heart muscle due to a sudden blockage in one or more coronary arteries. This can lead to a heart attack (myocardial infarction) or unstable angina (chest pain or discomfort that occurs when the heart muscle doesn't receive enough oxygen-rich blood). ACS requires immediate medical attention, as it can have serious and potentially life-threatening consequences.

angina
describes chest pain or discomfort that occurs when the heart muscle does not receive an adequate supply of oxygen-rich blood. It's typically caused by a narrowing or blockage in the coronary arteries, which are responsible for supplying blood to the heart. Angina can feel like pressure, tightness, or a squeezing sensation in the chest, and it may also radiate to the arms, neck, jaw, shoulder, or back. The pain often occurs during physical activity or emotional stress and tends to subside with rest or medication. Women often do not experience the same pain as men and have atypical chest pain which makes it more difficult to diagnose angina in women. It serves as a warning sign of an underlying heart condition and should be evaluated by a medical professional.

angina, unstable
is a more serious form of angina, characterised by chest pain or discomfort that occurs suddenly and unpredictably and rapidly becomes worse. Unlike stable angina, which is triggered by physical exertion or stress and tends to be consistent in its pattern, unstable angina can happen at rest or with minimal exertion. The pain is often more intense, prolonged, and not easily relieved by rest or medication. Unstable angina is a sign that a coronary artery is at high risk of becoming completely blocked and requires prompt medical attention, as it indicates an increased risk of a cardiovascular event.

angiogram
contrast (dye) injected into a patient's femoral or radial artery. This outlines the coronary arteries in exquisite detail, giving information about the location, the quality and nature of the plaque, the degree of stenosis and the size of the vessel affected. There are two types of coronary angiogram:

> **CT coronary angiogram** or a CTCA, a coronary computed tomography angiogram, which is non-invasive, and

> **'invasive' angiogram** as it requires a small tube to be passed from an artery in the arm or leg to the heart to inject dye directly into the arteries.

angiotensin II (AT2)
enzyme that works on the angiotensin II receptor and causes vasoconstriction – keeps up the blood pressure; dilates the kidney's efferent arteriole and so reduces filtration. The resultant fluid overload places a strain on the heart that could be detrimental to a heart in cardiac failure.

angiotensin II (AT2) **receptor**
drives much of the action within the renin-angiotensin-aldosterone system (RAAS), including the production of aldosterone

angiotensin II (AT2) receptor blocker (ARB)
acts directly on the AT2 receptor in the renin-angiotensin-aldosterone system (RAAS), releasing sodium and water, which then passes from the body as urine; lowers blood pressure, constricts efferent arteriole, lessens aldosterone production. Commonly used drugs are candesartan, telmisartan and valsartan. Should not be given with ACE inhibitors, although they are interchangeable.

angiotensin-converting enzyme (ACE)
the enzyme that converts angiotensin I (AT1) to angiotensin II (AT2)

angiotensin-converting enzyme (ACE) inhibitor
blocks the renin-angiotensin-aldosterone system (RAAS) – prevents the conversion of AT1 to AT2 – releasing sodium and water, which then passes from the body as urine. Used for patients whose hearts are not pumping well – hearts with reduced ejection fraction (HFrEF). Current commonly used drugs include enalapril, perindopril and ramipril. Should not be given with ARBs, although they are interchangeable.

anticoagulant
a blood thinner that slows down the formation of a clot and so helps reduce the risk of a clot forming; common agents are warfarin, heparin and non-vitamin K oral anticoagulants also called NOACS such as rivaroxaban, apixaban and dabigatran

antiplatelet
blood thinner that prevents blood components – platelets – from clumping together; helps reduce the risk of a clot forming; common agents are aspirin, ticagrelor and clopidogrel

arteries
the vessels of the body's circulation system that carry the blood away from the heart

> **aorta**
> the biggest artery of the body, takes the blood from the left ventricle as the blood begins its journey around the body. Coming from the aorta as it leaves the heart are
>
>> the **right coronary artery** (RCA) which provides blood to the surface of the heart, the area nearest the diaphragm, and
>>
>> the **left main coronary artery** (LM) which divides into
>>
>>> the **left anterior descending artery** (LAD) and provides blood to the anterior surface of the heart, the area nearest the chest wall, and
>>>
>>> the **circumflex artery** which provides blood to the back of the heart, the area nearest the spine
>
> **coronary arteries**
> are the first branches in the body's circulation system and supply oxygenated blood to the heart muscle
>
> **carotid arteries**
> a pair of major blood vessels in the neck that deliver blood to the brain and head
>
> **left internal mammary artery (LIMA)**
> an artery behind the sternum that supplies blood to the chest wall; considered a conduit of choice in coronary artery bypass graft (CABG) surgery. Also known as the internal thoracic artery (ITA).

radial artery
supplies blood to the forearm and the hand; can be used as the conduit in coronary artery bypass graft (CABG) surgery

arteries, layers
a healthy layer artery consists of three layers:

> an **inner** layer of endothelial cells – *tunica intima*, meaning inner coat
>
> a **middle** layer of smooth, muscle cells – *tunica media*, middle coat
>
> an **outer** layer of collagen – *tunic adventitia*, outside coat

aspirin
is the registered name for acetylsalicylic acid. Developed and manufactured by the German pharmaceutical company Bayer, it is the most widely used medical preparation in the world, with about 100 billion pills produced each year. Aspirin works by blocking the enzyme, cyclooxygenase, which alters production of prostaglandins, which then causes numerous impacts throughout the body.

associations
connected, joined or related to

atherosclerosis
the process of the gradual build-up of plaque in the arteries. Fatty deposits, cholesterol, and other substances build up within the walls of arteries, forming plaques that then narrow and harden the arteries, reducing blood flow to various parts of the body, including the heart, brain, and limbs.

atherosclerotic cardiovascular disease (ASCVD)
covers several conditions including coronary artery disease, cerebral and neck artery disease, and peripheral artery disease that result from atherosclerosis *(see above)*. It can lead to serious complications such as heart attacks, strokes, and other CV problems. Managing risk factors such as high blood pressure, high cholesterol, and a healthy lifestyle can help prevent and manage ASCVD.

atrial fibrillation (AF)
an 'irregularly irregular' heartbeat, characterised by the loss of the coordinated contraction of the top part of the heart, the atrial chambers, or atria. It affects the pumping capacity of the heart. The condition can be managed but not cured.

atrium
a pre-pumping chamber of the heart. There is an atrium on each side of the heart:

> the **right atrium** moves blood from the body through the right ventricle to the lungs,
>
> the **left atrium** moves blood from the lungs through the left ventricle into the body.

B

bariatric surgery
covers a set of weight-loss procedures designed to treat severe obesity when other weight loss methods have been unsuccessful. These surgeries aim to help individuals reduce their food intake, feel fuller faster, and absorb fewer calories from the food they eat.

beta-blockers
drugs frequently used to control the heart rate. They
- dampen the over-drive effect of the sympathetic nervous system which has nerve endings supplying the AV node, reducing the speed of electrical conduction from the atria to the ventricles and thus slowing the heart rate, and
- target the high density of beta receptors (specifically beta2 receptors) in the heart;
- improve mortality, morbidity and quality of life for people with reduced cardiac function

commonly used drugs are metoprolol, atenolol, carvedilol, bisoprolol, extended-release metoprolol and nebivolol

blood
the bodily fluid that transports oxygen and nutrients to the body and removes carbon dioxide and other waste. Among its components are platelets (which help in clot formation).

blood clot (thrombus)
a soft, thick lump comprising platelets and fibrin to prevent blood loss if a blood vessel is damaged. A clot can also form inside an artery or vein and stop or block the normal flow of blood. This situation can be very dangerous. If it dislodges and travels though the circulatory system, this is called embolization and can cause a major disaster within the body, such as stroke, pulmonary embolism, deep vein thrombosis (DVT), kidney failure or pregnancy complications.

blood flow restoration
procedures to restore or improve blood flow to blocked arteries that include the implantation of a stent/s or bypass grafting

blood pressure (BP)
refers to the force exerted by blood against the walls of arteries as the heart pumps the blood around the body. It is measured in millimetres of mercury (mmHg) and consists of two values: systolic (higher) and diastolic (lower) pressure. For instance, a reading of 120/80 mmHg indicates a systolic pressure of 120 and a diastolic pressure of 80. A BP reading helps assess cardiovascular health and the risk of various conditions:

> **diastolic** – is the lower value in a BP reading and represents the pressure in the arteries when the heart is at rest, filling with blood, between beats;

> **systolic** – the higher value in a BP reading and reflects the pressure in the arteries when the heart contracts and pumps blood into the circulation (the pressure during a heartbeat's peak force). Monitoring systolic BP is crucial for evaluating cardiovascular well-being.

body mass index (BMI)
is a measurement based on the height and weight of a person and is used to determine if a person is in a healthy weight range. It is calculated by dividing a person's weight in kilograms by the square of the person's height in meters. The resulting value indicates whether a person is underweight, normal weight, overweight, or obese. However, it does not consider factors such as muscle mass, bone density, and distribution of fat, so it's important to consider it alongside other health indicators.

C

calcium
is a mineral that can become a component of plaque and so end up in the arteries in the context of coronary artery disease. Its presence is used as an indicator of potential risk based on the coronary artery calcium (CAC) score.

calcium channel blocker
stops calcium from entering the cells of the heart and the arteries; used for high blood pressure, chest pain and irregular heartbeat; common agents include nifedipine and amlodipine (peripherally-active) and diltiazem and verapamil (centrally-active); agents best avoided in the presence of cardiac failure

carbohydrates
one of the three main macronutrients found in food, alongside proteins and fats. They are organic compounds made up of carbon, hydrogen, and oxygen atoms. Carbohydrates serve as a primary source of energy for the body. They are classified into simple and complex carbohydrates based on their chemical structure and how quickly they are digested and absorbed by the body.

cardiac arrest (*see* sudden cardiac arrest, SCA)

cardiac failure (CF)
also referred to as heart failure
is a condition in which the heart does not pump as well as it should, leading to a complex mix of a sick heart, maladapted responses to impaired circulation and fluid retention that further strains the heart into a downward spiral of deterioration

cardiac failure, acute
when the heart fails, acutely (suddenly, severely); a medical emergency

cardiac imaging
any method used to image the muscle, valves and arteries of the heart:

> **echocardiography** assesses size and dynamic function such as blood flow of muscle and valves
>
> **CT imaging** assesses the health and structure of the arteries in a non-invasive way
>
> **invasive angiography** provides the clearest picture of the narrowing of the arteries
>
> **magnetic resonance imaging** (MRI)/ **cardiac magnetic resonance** (CMR) assesses size and dynamic function such as blood flow of muscle and valves shows scarring within the heart and inflammation, in exquisite detail
>
> **nuclear medicine** assesses aspects of cellular function, blood flow and heart function; also used for stress testing

cardio-pulmonary resuscitation (CPR)
is an emergency lifesaving technique, of hard and fast chest compressions in association with mouth-to-mouth resuscitation, used when someone's breathing or heartbeat has stopped. Even if untrained and uncertain about what to do, it is always better to try something than to do nothing. The difference between doing something and doing nothing could be someone's life.

causations
factors/actions that cause the problem

cardiovascular disease (CVD)
general term for conditions affecting the heart or blood vessels; includes coronary heart disease, angina, heart attack, congenital heart disease, stroke and vascular dementia

cholesterol
a waxy, fat-like, water-insoluble organic substance that is an essential component of all animal (including human) cells. It is produced naturally in all cells in the body, especially in the liver and reproductive organs, and found also in food. The risk of developing heart disease rises and falls with the rise and fall of cholesterol levels in the blood. As high cholesterol does not lead to apparent symptoms, levels should be checked regularly through blood testing.

> **HDL** or 'good' cholesterol carries cholesterol away from the arteries and back to the liver to be broken down, and passed from the body as waste,
>
> **LDL** or 'bad' cholesterol is implicated in the build-up of plaque within the arteries, which can lead to blockages, preventing enough blood from flowing to the heart, and causing a heart attack.

coronary artery bypass graft (CABG)
a major surgical procedure used to treat coronary artery disease (CAD), in which part of a healthy vein or artery is used to divert blood around narrowed or clogged arteries to improve blood flow to the heart muscle

coronary artery calcium (CAC) **score**
based on a CT scan; has become the standard marker for indicating plaque build-up within the arteries (atherosclerosis)

coronary artery disease (CAD) or **coronary heart disease** (CHD)
the process of atherosclerosis, or plaque build-up, in the artery that leads to a narrowing of the artery and reduced blood flow. If left undetected, this can produce symptoms including angina and shortness of breath, and lead to a heart attack.

coronary atherosclerosis (*see* plaque)

COVID
is short for Coronavirus Disease 2019, an infectious disease caused by a novel coronavirus known as SARS-CoV-2. The virus was first identified in Wuhan, China, in December 2019, and it quickly spread globally, leading to a pandemic. COVID-19 primarily spreads through respiratory droplets and can cause a range of symptoms, including death, particularly in older adults and those with underlying health conditions.

D

dementia
is a general term used to describe a group of cognitive impairments that affect memory, thinking, reasoning, and other mental abilities to the extent that they interfere with daily life and functioning

depression
a common illness worldwide that is characterised by severe and prolonged low mood; is different to usual mood fluctuations and short-lived emotional responses to challenges in everyday life. The affected person can suffer greatly and function poorly. At worst, it can lead to suicide.

diabetes
is a chronic disorder that occurs when the body has difficulty regulating blood sugar (glucose) levels due to insufficient production of insulin, ineffective use of insulin, or a combination of both. Both forms of diabetes can lead to high blood sugar levels, which, if not properly managed, can cause various health complications over time, affecting the eyes, kidneys, nerves, heart, and blood vessels. Management involves monitoring blood sugar levels, adopting a healthy lifestyle, taking prescribed medications, and regular medical check-ups.

> **pre-diabetes** occurs when blood sugar levels are higher than normal but not yet high enough to be classified as type 2 diabetes. It serves as a warning sign that a person is at increased risk of developing diabetes in the future.
>
> **type 1** is a chronic condition in which the immune system mistakenly attacks and destroys the insulin-producing cells in the pancreas. Individuals with type 1 diabetes have little to no insulin production. It is often inherited and not preventable and is typically diagnosed in childhood or adolescence, although it can occur at any age.
>
> **type 2** is a chronic condition characterised by insulin resistance, where the body's cells do not respond effectively to insulin. Glugose (sugar) builds up in the bloodstream, leading to high blood sugar levels.

diuretic
medication to make a patient pass fluid – relieves congestion and reduces strain on the heart

diuretic, loop
medication that works by blocking the concentrating mechanisms within the loop of the renal tubule, the Loop of Henle; the most used drug is furosemide (frusemide)

E

echocardiogram (echo)
echo, sound, *cardio*, heart, *gram*, picture
a scan of the heart using ultrasound waves to acquire a picture. It gives information about the valves, the chambers of the heart and pressures within the heart.

electrocardiogram (ECG)
a trace of the electrical activity through the heart acquired by electrodes. It shows the rhythm of the heart. Features of an ECG can be used to determine the status of the heart muscle.

> **P wave**
> electrical activity in the atria, reflecting actual depolarization or the electrical flow. No P wave with chaotic electrical activity is the diagnostic thumbprint of atrial fibrillation.
>
> **QRS complex**
> created by the electrical impulses reflecting the depolarisation of the major muscle of the heart
>
> **T wave**
> the return of normal repolarization to the heart muscle ready for the next beat

exercise
physical activity that involves planned, structured, and repetitive movements of the body aimed at improving or maintaining physical fitness and overall health. Regular exercise offers numerous benefits for the body and mind.

extracorporeal membrane oxygenation (ECMO)
a machine, very similar to a bypass machine, that takes blood from the patient to transfer oxygen through a membrane outside the body to maintain oxygenation to the person; used for critically unwell patients with a good chance of recovery

F

familial hypercholesterolemia
a common genetically inherited condition in which the body produces too much cholesterol and cannot clear it. This causes early onset cardiovascular disease (before the age of 55 for men, and 60 women) and needs to be treated from an early age.

G

gliflozin
the sodium-glucose transport inhibitor (SGLT2 inhibitor) that
- works at the proximal tubule of the kidney, allowing salt and water to be lost through the urine; developed initially to aid diabetics
- reduces hospitalisations
- improves quality of life especially for diabetic patients with CF, and
- improves mortality

the first drug identified to provide benefit in cardiac failure was empagliflozin, while a 2019 report to the European Society of Cardiology showed that the drug, dapagliflozin, was a beneficial add-on therapy for cardiac failure patients already appropriately treated regardless of whether or not they had diabetes. The SGLTs-1 drugs are now included as routine therapy for patients with reduced ejection fraction cardiac failure.

glucagon-like peptide-1 receptor antagonist (GLP-1 RA)
a drug for diabetes that appears to reduce cardiac events; agents include semaglutide, dulaglutide and exenatide

glucose
a sugar; a vital source of energy for the body's cells, especially for the brain and muscles

H

Healthy Heart Network
a social media network founded by Warrick Bishop to promote heart health through education, helping people live as well as possible for as long as possible (https://healthyheartnetwork.com/index)

heart / heart muscle
a large muscle that pumps blood through the body
the term 'heart' usually refers to the entire organ responsible for pumping blood throughout the body. It includes the various components like the chambers, valves, and blood vessels. The 'heart muscle' specifically refers to the myocardium, which is the muscular tissue that makes up the walls of the heart's chambers. The heart muscle contracts and relaxes rhythmically to pump blood effectively. In short, the 'heart' encompasses the entire organ, while the 'heart muscle' refers to the muscular tissue within the heart's walls.

Heart 180
founded by Guy Leech to distribute world-leading brands of defibrillators. Heart 180's mission is to have a defibrillator with in 180 seconds of every Australian (https://heart180.com.au/)

heart attack
a non-medical expression. It is a layman's term referring to a myocardial infarction
myo, muscle, *cardio*, heart, *infarction*, death by lack of blood flow.

Most commonly, but not always, it is caused by the narrowing of the coronary arteries that can kill or requires some form of medical intervention – medication, time in hospital, balloons or stents, or coronary artery bypass grafting. There are two types of heart attack:

> **NSTEMI** a non-ST-Elevation Myocardial Infarction, in which the coronary artery is partially and temporarily blocked.

> **STEMI** a ST-Elevation Myocardial Infarction, in which the coronary artery is completely and permanently blocked.

The type of heart attack is determined by the results of the ECG. While the NSTEMI is the less serious of the two because less damage is done to the heart, it is still a serious condition that requires immediate diagnosis and treatment.

heart disease (*see* coronary artery disease)

Heart of the Nation
founded by Greg Page to promote the understanding and use of automated external defibrillators (AEDs) and cardio-pulmonary resuscitation (CPR) (https://www.heartofthenation.com.au/)

I

insulin
a hormone produced by the pancreas that helps regulate glucose levels in the bloodstream and allows cells to use glucose for energy

L

lipids
a diverse group of organic molecules that include fats, oils, hormones, and certain components of cell membranes. Lipids are hydrophobic, meaning they don't mix well with water. They play essential roles in energy storage, insulation, cellular structure, and signalling within the body. Lipids include triglycerides, phospholipids, and cholesterol.

> **cholesterol** (*see* cholesterol)

> **triglycerides** the most common fat in the body; can increase the chances of developing plaque in the arteries, leading to a higher risk of heart attack or stroke.

lipid profile
or cholesterol blood test measures lipids (fats) in the blood. Typically, it includes measurements of total cholesterol (TC), high-density lipoprotein (HDL) cholesterol, low-density lipoprotein (LDL) cholesterol, and triglycerides. It can also include TC to HDL ratio, lipoprotein (a) and the level of non-HDL. A lipid profile provides valuable information about an individual's cardiovascular health, helping to assess the risk of heart diseases and guiding preventive measures or treatment.

lipoproteins
particles comprised of protein and fat that carry cholesterol through the blood to the tissues and back from the tissues to the liver

> **lipoprotein (a)** – Lp(a) is an inherited lipoprotein that looks and behaves like LDL with a glycoprotein (apo a) attached to it but is more atherogenic (substances or conditions that promote the development or progression of atherosclerosis). It is an independent strong risk factor for heart disease and stroke.

lungs
paired, spongy organs located within the chest cavity, enclosed by the ribcage. They are essential components of the respiratory system, responsible for the exchange of oxygen and carbon dioxide between the air we breathe and the bloodstream.

M

Mediterranean-style diet
this style of eating emphasises whole fruits, vegetables, whole grains, lean proteins, and healthy fats. It is inspired by the traditional eating patterns of countries bordering the Mediterranean Sea and includes olive oil, nuts, and fish. It is known for its potential heart health benefits and balanced approach to nutrition.

mineralocorticoid
mineralo, mineral balance; *corticoids*, steroid-based hormones
hormone messengers that influence electrolyte and water balance in the body; the primary mineralocorticoid is aldosterone

mineralocorticoid blocker
can be used as a diuretic. If used in conjunction with a loop diuretic, particular care needs to be exercised around fluid balance and fluid loss, with regular blood testing and clinical assessment essential.

myocardium
myo, muscle, *cardium*, being of the heart
the muscle of the heart

> **myocardium, hibernating** (*see* viable heart muscle)
>
> **myocardial infarction**
> *infarction*, death from lack of blood flow
> medical term for 'heart attack'; no blood flow/oxygen supply to the heart muscle
>
> **myocardial ischemia**
> *ischemia*, lack of blood
> reduced blood flow/oxygen supply to the heart muscle

N

nodes
> **sinoatrial** (SA) node
> a cluster of specialised heart cells located in the top of the right atrium and it is where the electrical activity of the heart originates and drives the rhythm of the heart

atrioventricular (AV) **node**
a cluster of cells in the centre of the heart between the atria and ventricles that allows electrical communication; also acts as a gatekeeper, regulating the electrical impulses as they come from the atria and enter the ventricles

O

obesity
a medical condition characterised by excess body fat accumulation. It can result from a combination of genetic, environmental, and lifestyle factors. Obesity is often measured using body mass index (BMI) and is associated with increased health risks, such as heart disease, diabetes, and joint issues.

P

platelets
small particles in the blood needed for the formation of clots; activated when there is an irregularity within a blood vessel. They are an essential element of the body's defence against bleeding disorders; they help maintain the integrity of the circulatory system. On the negative side, they can contribute to the formation of unwanted blood clots within the arteries.

plaque (coronary atherosclerosis)

    calcified
    the amount of calcium in the plaque

    cholesterol-dominant / non-calcific / low attenuation plaque (LAP)
    the build-up of lipids (fats) within the plaque; increased lipid content is associated with less stability, a greater likelihood of rupture

    flow-limiting
    the artery becomes 'tight'; symptoms include chest pain or shortness of breath on exertion

    non-flow-limiting
    there is no perceived limit to the blood-flow; no warnings; death is sudden and unexpected

prevention

    primary
    treatment for a risk before an event

    secondary
    treatment to prevent another event/problem from occurring

prognosis / prognostic
the long-term outcome for the patient

R

rehabilitation, cardiac
aims at preventing a second occurrence or progression of the disease; involves physical, mental, and social aspects; to have the patient live as healthy and active a life for as long as possible. Cardiac rehabilitation should be considered an essential component of post heart attack life for all patients.

renal artery denervation
a relatively new blood pressure lowering procedure that ablates, or destroys, the nerves running along the outside of the renal artery to the kidney. The premise is that these nerves of the sympathetic nervous system play an important role in driving elevated blood pressure through kidney mechanisms. When overactive, they contribute to high blood pressure.

revascularisation
a procedure to re-establish or improve blood flow with the use of stents or coronary artery bypass grafting

rhythm

> **sinus** (normal)
> the healthy heart rhythm, which is controlled by the sinoatrial, or sinus, node, beating in asynchronistic and smooth manner
>
> **arrhythmia**
> when the synchronicity of the heartbeat breaks down

risk
refers to the probability that an individual might experience an event such as a heart attack based on certain factors including medical history, lifestyle choices, genetics, and overall health. The risk of a coronary artery event is defined as low, intermediate, or high:

> **low** a less than 10 per cent chance of a coronary event within 10 years
>
> **high** a greater than 20 per cent chance of an event within 10 years
>
> **intermediate** between 10 and 20 per cent of an event within 10 years.

S

smoking
is the act of inhaling and exhaling the smoke produced by burning tobacco or other substances, often through cigarettes, cigars, or pipes. Smoking releases a complex mixture of chemicals, including nicotine, into the respiratory system resulting in a range of adverse health effects, including the increased risk of cardiovascular disorders. Quitting smoking, or avoiding exposure to tobacco smoke, can significantly reduce health risks and improve overall well-being.

> **e-cigarettes** (electronic cigarettes) are one of several vaping devices now available (*see below*, vaping)
>
> **passive** refers to the inhalation of smoke by individuals who are not actively smoking themselves
>
> **tobacco smoke** its combination of harmful chemicals and toxins can lead to numerous health problems
>
> **vaping** uses battery-operated devices, such as e-cigarettes) that vaporise a liquid solution into an aerosol that is inhaled by the user. This aerosol typically contains nicotine, flavourings, and other chemicals. Vaping aims to mimic the act of smoking traditional cigarettes without involving combustion. Long-term health effects are being studied. Concerns exist about the appeal of this method of smoking to youth and non-smokers.

sodium-glucose transport inhibitor (SGLT2) (*see* gliflozin)

stenosis
narrowing

stent / stenting
a mechanical intervention for coronary artery disease in which an intravascular device (balloon) within a wire scaffold is inserted percutaneously (through the skin) and guided to the site of the narrowing. When the balloon is inflated, the artery is opened. When the balloon is removed, the wire scaffold remains to keep it open. The scaffold is called a stent.

stress test
a test of heart function that is used to diagnose coronary artery disease. It involves exercising the patient, or giving the patient medication to replicate exercise, to try to reproduce angina under investigation or unmask areas where there is a lack of blood flow to the heart.

stroke
a disruption of the blood supply to the brain leading to permanent loss of function

> **haemorrhagic** when a blood vessel ruptures and bleeds into the brain
>
> **ischemic** when a clot (also called thrombus) blocks an artery, leading to a lack of blood flow. Such clots often form in the large blood vessels in the neck, the carotid arteries, or in the heart because of atrial fibrillation

sublingual glyceryl trinitrate (GTN)
a spray under the tongue, to be used when a person experiences chest pain (angina); it is given with some caution; not to be used with Viagra

sudden cardiac arrest (SCA)
occurs when the electrical impulses of the heart malfunction, leaving the heart unable to pump blood to the body. The symptoms are immediate, with the person non-responsive and not breathing. It can happen to anyone at any time. The causes vary. Without immediate action (CPR and defibrillation), only a small percentage of sufferers survive.

T

thiazides
a mainstay of blood pressure therapy, they block the sodium (salt) retaining function of the distal convoluted tubule in the kidney (the resulting salt and water loss reduces blood volume and so lowers blood pressure) and lower blood pressure by dilating (relaxing or widening) the blood vessels

U

unstable angina (*see* angina, unstable)

V

valves
keep blood flowing through the heart in the right direction
(in order of blood flow)

> **tricuspid** a one-way valve between the right atrium and the right ventricle
>
> **pulmonary** a one-way valve between the right ventricle and the pulmonary circulation, which takes the blood to the lungs

mitral a one-way valve between the left atrium and the left ventricle

aortic a one-way valve between the left ventricle and the aorta, which is the main artery leading from the heart into the body

veins
low pressure blood vessels that mostly carry deoxygenated blood towards the heart. The ones that most concern us are:

IVC, inferior vena cava is one of two major veins that drains into the right atrium; it collects blood flowing below the heart

jugular vein carries blood from the brain, face and neck, and connects with the SVC to take the blood to the right atrium; a 'dipstick' for fluid pressure in the right atrium (the waveform of the jugular pulse is often visible in patients with a sick heart when sitting upright)

pulmonary veins are the exception, and the four pulmonary veins transfer oxygenated blood from the lungs to the left atrium of the heart

saphenous vein (the great saphenous vein, GSV) is the longest vein in the body; part of the vein, taken from the calf or thigh, is a commonly used medium in coronary artery bypass graft (CABG) surgery, with a 40-50 per cent failure rate after 10 years

SVC, superior vena cava is one of two major veins that drains into the right atrium; it collects blood flowing above the heart

ventricle
the main compression (pumping) chamber of the heart that pushes the blood through the body. There is a right and the left ventricle

right ventricle pumps the oxygen-poor blood into the lungs

left ventricle (the main pumping chamber of the heart) pumps oxygen-rich blood into the body

viable heart muscle (*see* myocardium, hibernating)

W

walking
called the 'wonder drug' by the Heart Foundation (Australia), this fundamental form of human movement offers numerous health benefits including cardiovascular fitness, improved joint mobility, stress reduction, and mental relaxation

INDEX

A

acute coronary syndrome 43, 46, 213

AED *(see defibrillator)*

angina (fn9) 28, 43, 46, 55, 67, 79, 125, 168, 179, 213, 218, 225

    unstable 46, 200, 213

angiogram (angiography) 20, 21, 175, 176, 186, 213

    CT coronary angiogram (CTCA) 8, (fn2) 28, 147, 148, 149, 213, 217

    'invasive' angiogram 20, 23, 24, 146, 153, 213

angiotensin I 124, 214

angiotensin II (AT2) 124, 213, 214

angiotensin II (AT2) receptor 213

angiotensin II (AT2) receptor blocker (ARB) 124, 168, 214

angiotensin-converting enzyme (ACE) 214

angiotensin-converting enzyme (ACE) inhibitor 124, 152, 168, 214

anticoagulant/s 168, 214

antiplatelet 168, 214

artery/ies 21, 23, 25, (fn2, fn3) 28, 31, 32, 36, 37, 41, 42, 43, 44, 46, 51, 55, 56, 59, 67, 70, 72, 79, 95, 118, 119, 120, 125, 136, 137, 138, 140, 141, 142, 143, 144, 145, 146, 146, 148, 149, 152, 154, 155, 156 157, 162, 168, 177, 178, 187, (fn84) 195, 200, 213, 214-215, 216, 217, 218, 221, 223

    arteriole/s (efferent) 39, 125, 213, 114

    aorta 34, 35, 36, 119, 120, 214, 226

    carotid 39, 214, 225

    chest wall 36, 178, 214

    circumflex 36, 37, 142, 151, 214

    coronary 15, 17, 24, 32, 36, 37, 40, 41, 43, 52, 55, 145, 146, 147, 151, 167, 178, 179, 200, 211, 213, 214, 221

    hardening of the 67, 117, 215

    layer/s of the 42, 43, 215

    left anterior descending (LAD) 36, 37, 206, 214

    left internal mammary (LIMA) 178, 214

    left main coronary (LM) 36, 179, 214

    leg/s 67, 125, 167, 179

    narrow/ed/ing 70, 79, 124, 137, 144, 149, 151, 152, 179, 200, 213, 215, 217, 218, 221, 225

    neck 167, 214, 215, 225

    pulmonary 34, 35

    radial (arm) 178, 179 213, 215

    right coronary (RCA) 36, 37, 140, 142, 214

    vertebral 39

    walls of the 42, 117, 125, 138, 155, 215, 216

aspirin 18, 49, 55, 58, 71, 73, 75, 95, 141, 152, 158, 162, 163-170, 214, 215

associations 57, 59-60, 162, 215

atherosclerosis 8, 11, 45, 67, 70, 79, 145, 156, 168, 215, 218, 222

atherosclerotic cardiovascular disease (ASCVD) 117, 130, 215

atrial fibrillation (AF) 9, 33, 70, 71, 95, 118, 119, 123, 168, 210, 211, 212, 215, 219, 225, 237

atrium (right, left)/atria 31, 32, 33, 34, 35, 38, 39, 215, 216, 219, 222, 223, 225, 226

B

bariatric surgery 100, 101, 102, 215,

beta-blockers 124, 168, 216,

blood (blood is used extensively throughout the book)

    clot/thrombus 38, 41, 48-49, 50, 53, 95, 137, 151, 164, 206, 214, 216, 225

    flow restoration 216

    stream 42, 44, 49, 70, 71, 85, 111, 161, 164, 219, 221, 222

blood pressure (BP) 42, 55, 56, 57, 60, 70, 71, 75, 77, 79, 85, 86, 88, 95, 96, 99, 100, (fn47) 102, 113, 116, 117-126, 128, 130, 132, 133, 136, 137, 143, 150, 156, 166, 168, 188, 213, 214, 215, 216, 217, 224, 225

body mass index (BMI) 101, (fn45) 102, 216, 223

C

calcium 9, 45, 53, (fn17) 64, 72, 124, 145, 146, 147, 148, 149, 217, 223

calcium score (*see coronary artery calcium score*)

calcium channel blockers 124, 168, 217

capillaries 38, 39

carbohydrate/s 70, 71, 85, 95, 97, (fn47) 102, 107, 109, 110, 111, 112, (fn58) 116, 128, 132, 152, 217

cardiac arrest (*see sudden cardiac arrest*)

cardiac failure (CF) 9, 71, 95, 118 119, 132, 133, 211, 212, 213, 217, 220, 237

cardiac imaging 52, 217

    angiography 8, 147, 153, 217

    CT imaging 8, 37, 139, 152, 217

    echocardiography/gram 151, 153, 219

    electrocardiogram (ECG) 20, 151, 152, 219, 221

cardio-pulmonary resuscitation (CPR) 51, (fn84) 195, 203, 206, 207, 209, 217, 221, 225

causations 59, 217

cardiovascular disease (CVD) 26, (fn13) 28, 67, 70, 77, 78, 79, (fn31) 82, 87, 92, 93, (fn35) 94, 110, (fn48, fn49) 115, (fn51) 116, 129, 135, 166, (fn79) 170, 200, (fn85) 201, 212, 218, 220

    Australian Cardiovascular Disease Risk Calculator 139, 143, 157

cholesterol 8, 10, 12, 18, 20, 22, 38, 43, 44, 45, 53, 55, 56, 58, 59, 60, 61, 71, 72, 75, 79, 85, 86, 100, 107, (fn51) 116, 121, 128, 130, 135, 136, 138, 139, 140, 141, 143, 146, 148, 150, 154, 155-162, 168, 205, 215, 218, 220, 221, 222, 223

    HDL 44, 113, 139, 141, 143, 155, 156, 157, 158, 160, 218, 221

    LDL 43, 44, 45, 53, 72, 88, 105, 106, 139, 141, 143, 145, 1 55, 1 56, 157, 158, 161, 218, 221, 222

    (*also see lipids*)

coronary artery bypass graft/ing (CABG)/bypass surgery 17, 21, 23, 24, 26, 27, 55, 175, 178, 179, 187, 198, 191, 214, 215, 218, 221, 224, 226

coronary artery calcium score (CAC)/scoring 140, 141, 144, 145, 146, 147, 149, 158, 159, 195, 217, 218

coronary artery disease (CAD) or coronary heart disease (CHD) 8, 18, 20, 21, 43, 46, 56, 60, 67, 74, 95, 99, 117, 136, 139, 145, 152, 157, 158, 175, 191, 200, (fn85) 201, 203, 215, 217, 218,

coronary atherosclerosis (*see plaque*)

COVID 18, 176, 184, 194, 218

D

defibrillator/s (automated external defibrillator – AED) 12, 51, 203, 204, 205, 207, 209, 221, 236

dementia 74, 77, 96, 119, (fn69) 34, 218

depression 69, 85, 88, 90, 91, 93, (fn37) 94, 129, 173, 218

diabetes 55, 56, 71, 75, (fn21) 75, 77, 86, (fn35) 94, 95, 96, 170, 111, 112, 121, 127-134, 136, 137, (fn78) 170, 219, 220, 223

    pre-diabetes 71, 96, 135, 219

    type 1 127, 128, 129, 219

    type 2 71, 84, 85, 93, 99, 101, 127, 128, 129, 130, 131, (fn75) 134, 135, 219

    Diabetes Australia 129, (fn70, fn71, fn73) 134, 212

diuretic/s 168, 124, 219, 222

E

echocardiogram (echo)/ electrocardiogram (ECG) *(see cardiac imaging)*

exercise/s/ing 12, 19, 20, 39, 55, 59, 60, 61, 69, 71, 73, 75, 82, 83-86, 87, 88, 89, 91, 93, (fn32, fn36, fn37) 94, 96, 98, 114, 117, 121, 130, 136, 137, 146, 151, 152, 153, 156, 160, 172, 173, 185, 205, 219, 225

extracorporeal membrane oxygenation (ECMO) 178, 182, 191, 220

F

familial hypercholesterolemia 8, 135, 155, 220

fibrin 38, 47, 48, 49, 216

G

gliflozin 131, 132, (fn75) 134, 220

glucagon-like peptide-1 receptor antagonist (GLP-1 RA) 99, (fn47) 102, 131, 132-133, 220

glucose 99, 110, 111, 128, 131, 132, 133, (fn75) 134, 219, 220, 221, 224

H

Healthy Heart Network 9, 25, 91, (fn39, fn43) 94, 193, 194, (fn83) 195, 204, 205, 209, (fn9) 209, 210, 220

heart muscle 26, 40, 41, 43, 46, 47, 50, 51, 53, 70, 148, 152, 178, 200, 213, 214, 218, 219, 220, 222, 226

Heart 180 (fn82) 195, 203, 204, 221

heart attack/s 3, 8, 9, 15, 17, 21, 22, 24, 25, 26, 27, (fn12) 28, 40, 41, 43, 44, 50, 51, 52, 53, 55, 56, 57, 58, 60, 61, 62, 64, 67, 68, 70, 71, 72, 74, 75, 79, 80, 81, 82, 85, 90, 92, 93, 95, 103, 104, 105, 106, 112, 117, 118, 119, 123, 126, 129, 136, 145, 149, 151, 153, 154, 155, 156, 160, 164, 165, 166, 167, 168, 169, (fn81) 170, 171, 172, 174, 175, 176, 179, 187, 189, 193, 194, (fn84) 195, 199, 200, 207, 211, 211, 212, 213, 215, 218, 221, 222, 223, 224, 237

heart disease *(see coronary artery disease)*

Heart of the Nation 208, 209, 221

hypertension 96, 116, 117, 120, 125, (fn67) 126, 128

I

insulin 85, 86, 97, 99, 100, 127-134, 219, 221

L

lipid/s/profile/lowering 8, 10, 11, 45, 139, 141, 143, 148, 152, 157, 158, 161, 221, 223, 236

    cholesterol *(see cholesterol)*

    triglycerides 139, 141, 143, 156, 157, 158, 160, 121

    lipoproteins 43, 44, 45, 139, 141, 143, 155, 155, 157, 158, 221, 222

    lipoprotein (a) – Lp(a) 10, 156, 221, 222

lungs 31, 35, 38, 39, 40, 46, 79, 179, 182, 188, 189, 215, 222, 225, 226

M

Mediterranean-style diet 104, 105, 106, 107, 112, 114, (fn48, fn 49) 115, (fn51) 116, 222

mineralocorticoid/s/blocker 44, 222

myocardium 153, 220, 222, 226

O

obesity (fn35) 94, 94, 95-102, 127, 128, 135, 215, 223

P

peripheral vascular disease (PVD) 67, 79, 167, 169

platelets 38, 45, 47, 48, 49, 55, 164, 165, 214, 216, 223

plaque (coronary atherosclerosis) (fn2) 28, 37, 43-45, 46, 47, 50, 51, 53, 56, 67, 72, 117, 136, 137, 138, 140, 145, 146, 147, 148, 149, 151, 155, 156, 159, 162, 164, 168, 200, 213, 215, 217, 218, 221, 223

    calcified 47, 53, 72, 147, 223

    cholesterol-dominant / non-calcific / low attenuation plaque (LAP) 148-149, 223

    flow-limiting 46, 47, 53, 223

    non-flow-limiting 46, 47, 50, 53, 136, 137, 151, 223

prevention 3, 52, 64, 71, 85, 126, 130, 133, (fn69) 134, 138, 172, 174, 194, 223

    primary 56, 58, 64, 72, 73, 104-105, 107, (fn 48, fn 49) 115, 130, 136, 137, 145, 165, 166, 167, 223

    secondary 55, 56, 64, 72, 73, 88, 104, 105-106, 107, 136, 167, 201, 223

R

rehabilitation, cardiac 9, 25, 26, 27, 43, 91, (fn 34, fn39, fn43) 94, 171, 186, 205, (fn9) 209, 210, 211, 212, 223, 237

renal artery denervation 125, 224

S

smoke/ing/er 22, 24, 55, 56, 57, 60, 61, 68, 75, 76, 77-82, (fn25, fn28, fn29) 82, 87, 88, 117, 121, 135, 136, 156, 224

    e-cigarettes 78, 79, 80, 82, (fn24) 82, 224

    passive 68, 79, 80, 82, 224

    tobacco 78, 79, (fn25) 82, 224

    vaping 68, 77, 79, 224

sodium-glucose transport inhibitor (SGLT2) (*see gliflozin*)

stenosis 20, (fn2) 28, 149, 213, 225

stent/stenting 12, 20, 21, 23, 26, 27, 43, 55, 95, 123, 153, 179, 194, 211, 216, 221, 224, 225

stress test/s/ing 20, 136, 137, 141, 142, 146, 150-153, 217, 225

sudden cardiac arrest (SCA) 50, 51, (fn15) 53, 193, (fn84) 195, 203, 204, 205, 206, 207, 208, 209, (fn89) 209, 217, 225

U

unstable angina (*see angina, unstable*)

V

valves (tricuspid, pulmonary, mitral, aortic) 32, 33, 35, 39, 40, 217, 219, 220, 225

vein/s 31, 32, 33, 34, 35, 39, 125, 148, 177, 178, 185, 188, 216, 218, 226

ventricle/s (left, right) 31, 32, 34, 35, 36, 38, 39, 119, 179, 214, 215, 216, 223, 225, 226

W

walk/ed/ing 19, 22, 25, 69, 70, 83, 84, 85, 86, 88, (fn33, fn38) 94, 98, 103, 114, 151, 183, 185, 189, 205, 226

ACKNOWLEDGEMENTS AND THANKS

The production of a book such as *10 Commandments of Heart Health Explained* is not a mere chance happening or a piece of serendipitous luck. Without many individuals' support, inspiration, talent, knowledge and experience, this book would have remained a promising concept poised for realisation.

So, I wish to acknowledge and thank my collaborator and co-author, colleague, and friend, **Karam Kostner**, a world-renowned lipid expert from Brisbane, Queensland, who contributed insightful perspectives and an astute viewpoint to the book's contents. Thanks are also extended to my **colleagues,** whom I hold in the highest regard, and who generously took time from their busy schedules to provide professional feedback and friendly encouragement. I'd also like to credit the **individuals** who contributed to the guideline papers accompanying this book. These guideline documents are significant works carried out by dedicated colleagues who volunteer their time to improve medical care.

I am grateful to my cardiac **patients** who, over the years, have added to the collective experience that forms the foundation upon which I have built this book, and especially to those whose case studies are used throughout its pages, bringing the often complex medical theory into the realm of lived reality.

Although he is not my patient, I am thankful to international surf champion **Guy Leech** for the foreword to *10 Commandments*. The sudden cardiac death of a 'fit and healthy' close friend changed his life so that now he is on a mission to have a defibrillator within 180 seconds of every Australian. His firsthand encounter with SCD and the subsequent transformative motivation it sparked brings an urgency that these pages would not otherwise have had.

Sharp-eyed practitioners of precision **John Harbinson** and **David Thomas** gave valuable and honest man-in-the-street comments.

Additionally, I have the backing of several exceptionally adept technical experts who put the words, graphics and pages together: designer and artist

Cathy McAuliffe, master of the computer **Beverly Waldie**, marketeer **John North** and his team, and my single-minded and passionate writing partner **Penny Edman**. Each brings skill, commitment, and eagerness to the work.

I am deeply grateful to these close associates, my partner **Chelle** and my supportive family, and everyone else involved in the production of *10 Commandments of Heart Health Explained*.

Warrick Bishop
Hobart, Australia
January 2024

BEHIND THE SCENES

writer – **Penelope Edman** is a freelance writer, editor, high performance coach and photographer based in Hobart, Tasmania, Australia. After beginning her print journalism career in Bundaberg, Queensland, in the late 1970s, she moved to Hobart in 1991. She is an Australasian award-winning journalist and editor, and her articles and photographs have been published throughout Australia and internationally.

She authored four non-fiction books before assisting Dr Bishop with *Have You Planned Your Heart Attack?*, *Atrial Fibrillation Explained*, *Cardiac Failure Explained*, *Cardiac Rehabilitation Explained* and now, also in association with Dr Kostner, *10 Commandments of Heart Health Explained*.

Her continuous engagement with the material contained in these books inspires her to maintain vigilance over her own heart health by addressing modifiable risks. Moreover, she motivates her family and friends to follow suit.

www.ingramcontent.com/pod-product-compliance
Lightning Source LLC
Chambersburg PA
CBHW062057290426
44110CB00022B/2622